The myth of perfection in childbirth

For Niek
The wind beneath my wings.

Special thanks to Robbie Zeins,
for making this book possible.

Translation: Ayesha Desousa
Illustrations: Dik Klut
Photograph: Anouk De Kleermaeker
Design: Niek de Bruijn

© Diana Koster, 2016
English edition: Uitgeverij Lannoo nv, Tielt

www.lannoo.com

D/2017/45/156 – NUR 851/770
ISBN 978 94 014 4372 2

DIANA KOSTER

The myth of perfection in childbirth

The impact of a difficult birth on your life
and what you can do about it.

LANNOO

Contents

Introduction

In my practice – first as a midwife and later as a coach for women – I have found that childbirth deeply affects the life of a woman and her partner. Fortunately, the effect is usually a positive one. Many people declare that the day of the birth of their child is one of the most beautiful days of their lives.

However, giving birth can also be a negative experience, even if you "get something wonderful out of it", namely a healthy baby. In fact, this makes it extra difficult to explain that your birth experience has left you with a bleak feeling. It is as if you are undervaluing or snubbing your child. You may be seen as a bore if you cannot let go of painful memories of the birth, and feel you need to talk about them, a year or several years after it happened, while, in the meantime, your child has learned to walk, speak or is even going to school.

You might be concerned that you are the only person who recalls her birth experience in a negative way. Perhaps you have the impression that every woman, except you, has a trouble-free birth; that every woman, except you, is capable of giving birth; that for every woman, except you, giving birth was among the best moments of her life. You believe there is something wrong with you. Nothing, however, is further from the truth. Research shows that almost a quarter of women giving birth for the first time have unpleasant feelings about their experience three years later.

For women having a second or third child, that number goes down to one in eight. You are certainly not the only one (on the contrary!), for whom childbirth was disappointing, whose experience was more a nightmare than a dream, and for whom birthing your child feels "unfinished", even long after delivery.

This book contains many childbirth accounts as well as practical exercises you can do in order to process the negative birth experience. You will find that you are not the only woman to experience "unusual" feelings since giving birth: feelings of sadness, depression, anxiety or irritability. Perhaps you feel you were somehow a failure during the birth. This book will help you transform the feeling of failure to a feeling of being merely disappointed that it didn't go completely according to plan. This transformation will make a world of difference for you and for your baby.

Consider the metaphor in which your system was "struck by lightning" while giving birth and that lightning, perhaps now for years, has stayed in your body. You can do something about this! And it is relatively easy to do. You don't need to keep the lightning in your body any longer. You don't deserve this burden, and neither do your relationships with your partner or your baby. The exercises in this book will help you reduce, and ultimately eliminate, the lightning from your system. I hope the anecdotes in this book will spark some recognition and prompt you to take action.

If you have bought or received this book and you are pregnant for the first time, please put it away for the moment and read it only after you have given birth, if you feel that your birth experience is still "unfinished". Some of the birth stories in this book are distressing and are not recommended if you are expecting for the first time. They may make you more anxious, and this would not be beneficial to you or your baby.

"I wish this book had existed four years ago. My friends and family seemed to be pushing the joy of motherhood down my throat, while, to me, the delivery felt more like a landslide or even an earthquake. The world kept turning and I felt like I had fallen off it since the birth. Yes, I had a beautiful daughter, but when I looked at her, I longed for my uncomplicated previous life, before she entered it. I yearned to be able to go where I wanted, to eat out when I felt like it, to meet up with friends. Now she was taking up most of the room in my life, my head, my heart, my time. The sense of responsibility all day, every day, was crushing. Just last year – three years after my daughter's birth – I realised that my sense of responsibility had been negatively affected by my birth experience. I had always been the responsible type; I was the eldest of four children, where the youngest was disabled and therefore needed the most attention.

"Julie's birth hurled me into a super-responsible mode. I wanted to do everything as well as possible but that just made me freeze up. I tried to keep all the balls in the air but they kept slipping out of my hands. The coaching sessions helped me link my freezing up and excessive sense of responsibility to my birth experience. Once I became aware of that connection I was able to work on becoming the old Maria again. I achieved this after a few coaching sessions and by using a number of the exercises in this book. We're now a year on and I can attest that I am much stronger, having made it through this 'battle'. I am currently six months pregnant with our second child. I feel self-confident, secure in my relationship with my partner and well prepared for the birth and for the time after it. Far from being anxious, I am even a little curious about how it's going to be." (Maria, 26 years old)

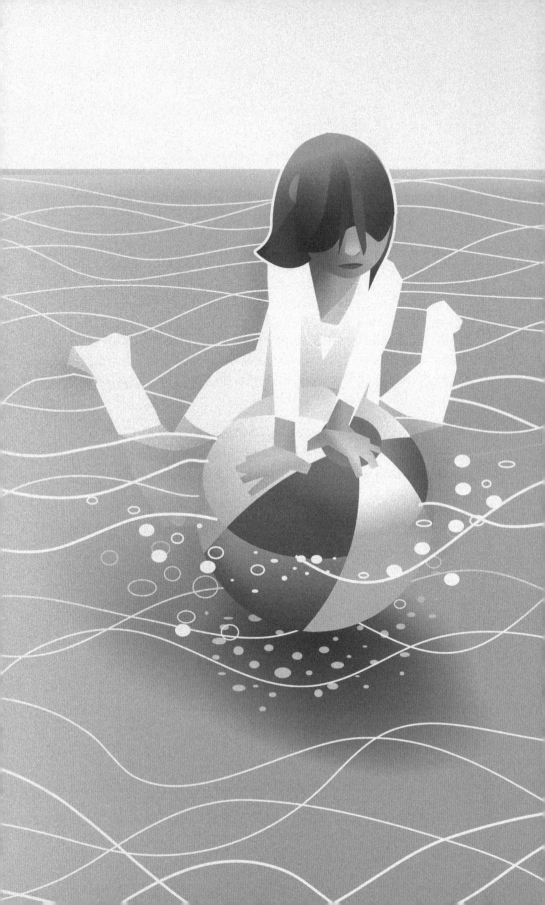

CHAPTER 1

To have a child,
a dream come true?

Having a child is a major life event: all-affecting and life-changing. The arrival of this little 2.7-kilo human bundle can turn your life upside down. There is the part of your life before you had a child and the part that began when you became a parent. These two phases in your life are impossible to compare and sometimes, unfortunately, impossible to reconcile.

It helps to have other people in your life who are going through the same phase. As new parents you can offer mutual support and learn from one another's experiences. It doesn't help if you are (or seem to be) the only one in your circle whose birth experience was far from perfect. That may give you the idea that your friends are unable to understand that you are still suffering from the effects of it.

The act of giving birth and the way you process the experience are very personal things. Perhaps on paper – and according to the midwife's or gynaecologist's report – your delivery was "spontaneous and without complications", while for you it feels like it was anything but straightforward. Your own experience of it was completely different. Some women can easily explain what made their delivery unpleasant, while others, such as Kim, find it much harder to put their finger on it.

"I couldn't understand it. Throughout my pregnancy I was radiant. I had prepared myself for labour. Within ten hours I had a beautiful and much-desired baby boy, without the need for an epidural, ventouse or forceps. I had – and have – the most wonderful husband in the world. Our parents are all healthy and couldn't wait for the chance to pamper and adore their first grandchild. I thought I would be over the moon and enormously proud to have given birth, but instead I found myself worrying about the whole episode.

Going through labour was so much more intense than I had ever imagined. Although the doctors said I had had a good delivery, for me it didn't feel 'good'. Precisely what didn't feel right, I couldn't put into words. Whenever I thought about my labour, I broke out into a sweat and my thoughts became completely blocked.

In contrast, my husband found it a hugely positive experience, 'the most beautiful of his life', and he couldn't understand why it made me so unhappy. In fact, I couldn't understand it myself. I became afraid of going to sleep, terrified I would have another nightmare about the birth and wake up bathed in sweat.

My first assignment from the coach was to write my birth story and read it out loud. I felt like I was writing about somebody else, as if I were retelling someone else's story – very strange. My coach asked if there was an exact moment I absolutely did NOT want to remember. Immediately an image sprang to mind, of needing to throw up while I was pushing the baby out. As soon as that image was in my mind, I had a gagging reflex and my eyes filled with tears.

The worst moment was when I threw up on myself and the nurse helped me out of my shirt. I can still remember the acrid smell when I think of it. I didn't have another shirt with me and both the doctor and the nurse told me it didn't matter, that plenty of women gave birth in the nude. But to me it did matter, and I didn't say so because I didn't want to appear childish or a prude.

I lay there, naked, on my back in bed, helpless and defenceless with strangers walking around the room and with bits of vomit in my hair, trying to give birth. It was dreadful! So unlike me! I felt so vulnerable, so exposed, as if I had been placed naked on a stage. Why did nobody think to drape a towel or a sheet over me? Why didn't I say anything? Why didn't my husband do anything? I couldn't control my sobbing when I thought back to that awful image.

In an exercise I replayed that part of the birth. In my version, I asked for the vomit to be wiped out of my hair and for my body to be covered with a sheet. In my version, this was done straight away and it felt much better. This simple exercise made me feel strong again. The delivery now felt right and I have not had the physical reactions or nightmares since then. Odd, isn't it?" (Kim, 32 years old)

In subsequent pregnancies, your expectations of labour can be coloured by your previous birth experience. While this previous experience can be positive, it can also be negative. In this case you may take a negative attitude or negative expectations into the new pregnancy, which increase the chance of you having a negative, unpleasant or disappointing birth once again.
The aim of this book is to help you process that initial negative experience so that your feelings about the birth and your baby are neutral and will not taint future deliveries.

The need to understand and to be understood

In my coaching sessions I find that most clients mainly have the need to understand and to be understood. They want to understand exactly what happened, why the midwife or gynaecologist chose to do (or not to do) certain things. They want to know how the baby was positioned in the pelvis and how he or she was born, why they needed a C-section or ventouse, and so on. Do not be afraid to ask your midwife or doctor these questions. I often use a baby doll and a scale model of a pelvis to explain precisely what happened during a birth. Sometimes parents are told the baby *"was not well positioned"*, but do not know what that meant in concrete terms.
Women also want to be understood; they want their feelings and doubts recognised. They yearn for recognition of what they went through during labour; recognition that things could have been done differently with hindsight; that what they went through wasn't trivial and that it's okay to have negative feelings when they recall the experience. Recognition that it's completely normal to feel the way they're feeling and that not everybody – far from it – is on cloud nine following childbirth.
Many mothers need (a lot of) time to adjust and do not have an immediate bond with their baby. It's absolutely normal to yearn for a time when there was no baby. They're so very tired now that they're mothers. It is very important that they feel that their family, friends and medical professionals understand

their own experience, thoughts and feelings. During the first coaching session I often hear my clients sigh with relief: *"So I'm not crazy?"* or *"So you don't think it's crazy that I feel this way?"* To which I reply: *"No, you're definitely not crazy. I understand that you're angry, afraid, sad. I understand from your story that that birth was a frightening and disappointing experience for you and I feel sorry for you."* It is normal and understandable to have powerful feelings after an intense childbirth experience. Unfortunately, when new mothers speak of their negative birth experience, their emotions are often discounted or played down:

- *"But, you got something wonderful out of it, didn't you? Your baby is healthy and well."*
- *"What did you expect, that childbirth would be easy? That you would just be able to do it?"*
- *"I know someone for whom it was much worse; she was in labour for more than 24 hours."*
- *"I can't believe you let that happen! You are normally so in control!"*
- *"It doesn't seem like you to have needed an epidural. I was sure you would manage without. I thought you were the sporty type."*

These remarks are obviously unhelpful. Far from being supportive, they reinforce your conviction that there is something wrong with you, that you've failed. A listening ear is the greatest gift somebody can offer you when you're trying to process a distressing experience. Ask those around you to simply listen to your story, your experience – over and over, until it has lost its sharp edges. Without interrupting and without sharing their own story and experiences – just to listen!

And when it's your turn to visit a friend, colleague or sister who has just given birth, listen to her story and her experience; don't wander off immediately into your own birth story.

Doctors and midwives are only human

Just listening and allowing people to tell their story is often enough to help the process of acceptance on its way.

When a woman recalls the delivery with her doctor or midwife, the medical professional can sometimes (unintentionally and even unconsciously) become defensive. Doctors and midwives usually do their utmost to give women a positive childbirth experience. If they are unsuccessful in this, they are often also troubled by it. Because of this, they can feel attacked when faced with questions about the decisions they made during the procedure. If a woman asks if things could have been handled differently, this might be interpreted by the medical staff as if the patient is challenging their knowledge, skill or effort. If somebody feels they are being attacked, a natural response is to become defensive (see the Drama Triangle theory in Chapter 8).

Moreover some medical staff find it difficult to put themselves in another's shoes. From their point of view – compared with other deliveries and from a medical perspective – a birth might be "without complications". From the point of view of the new parents, however, who are experiencing childbirth for the first time, it might be completely different. If, during the postnatal meeting, both parties stick stubbornly to their own standpoint ("routine" for the doctor; "a one-off, very intense and deeply moving event" for the parents), it is impossible to find common understanding. In such cases, parents don't feel their concerns have been taken seriously or they feel that the medical professionals are trying to protect one another.

The fear of complaints being filed against them sometimes plays a role too for doctors and midwives. They believe that it is unwise to agree with clients' concerns; that this would be "asking for trouble". In reality, the risk is small: the majority of complaints do not concern technical decisions taken during labour, but the personal treatment the parents experienced. Parents who feel their opinions have been heard and understood, and who are satisfied with the explanation given during the postnatal discussion as to why certain procedures were chosen and what, with hindsight, could have been done differently, usually do not file a complaint.

"The postnatal discussion did not go as I had hoped. I told the midwife that I had felt abandoned during labour. I found that difficult to express. Unfortunately, she immediately became defensive, saying that I had to understand I was not her only patient and that that particular day had been exceptionally busy. She still had ten newborn visits to carry out and she had been on duty for 24 hours. I felt as though she was not listening to me again, not taking me seriously again. I had been looking for understanding but instead it turned into an argument of who was right and who was wrong. During the birth I had begged her to stay with me because my husband, who was even more nervous than I was, could not offer me enough support. In spite of this, she left me alone, saying she would be back soon, at three o'clock, but only reappearing a few hours later. I had lain, focusing on the clock and waiting for her. Later on, she told me she wouldn't leave me again but then she went to check on another patient and only returned an hour later. Even in the postnatal meeting she was unable to put herself in my shoes but did expect me to try to understand her situation. It felt like a slap in the face all over again. For my next pregnancy I went to a different midwife practice."
(Merrill, 34 years old)

Fortunately, the postnatal meeting is increasingly a useful platform for new parents to begin to process their negative experience. Medical professionals are well intentioned. For them, childbirth has become so commonplace that they do not always realise that they sometimes need to provide extra clarification. Perhaps there was no time during the delivery to give detailed explanations because the doctor or midwife had to act quickly. Perhaps the experience was so overwhelming for the parents that they simply didn't hear the explanation. If you feel the need to talk about your birth experience, there is no need to wait until the postnatal check, which usually takes place six

weeks after the birth; you can make an earlier appointment.
Do specify, however, that you would like an appointment with
the doctor or midwife who was present during your delivery
and ask for an extra-long meeting so that they have a chance to
answer all your questions.

"During the postnatal discussion – which she purposely scheduled
at the end of her shift – the midwife made a lot of time for us. She
let me recount the whole birth again. She nodded and made notes.
She listened. She then came back to the points we apparently had
misunderstood or not understood at all and explained them again.
We were given the opportunity to ask all our questions and, by the
end of the meeting, we finally understood exactly what had happened:
why it had become an emergency situation, why our baby and I had
to travel in separate ambulances, why my baby was not allowed to
stay with me. The midwife said she had explained this at the time of
the delivery and again in the week after the birth. Curiously, we had
no memory of this; it was as if we were hearing it for the first time.
Only now, six weeks after the birth, were we in a position to absorb
the information. I believe that that meeting, which must have lasted
an hour, was the turning point for us. After it, we began to feel better
emotionally. The midwife phoned us again a couple of weeks later to
ask if we had any more questions or if anything was still unclear and
if we needed an additional meeting. What a service!"
(Elisabeth, 31 years old)

Feelings need to be felt

When calling to mind your birth experience, it is not the
objective medical report of the delivery that is important, but
your own subjective experience of it. You need those around
you to understand that the birth was a painful experience for
you. This recognition can help you process the event. Use the
postnatal meeting to ask about what, when and why things
happened. Do you have all the information you need?

Do you want to know more about the process of childbirth or the complications you had? Do you feel that the interventions taken were unnecessary or, on the contrary, that the doctors didn't take steps that they should have? Getting answers to these questions helps you to fill in the missing pieces of the puzzle.

If giving birth was an intense event for you, it would have summoned up intense emotions. These emotions need to be felt, rather than to be pushed down. I like to use a metaphor to describe this process. Imagine a beach ball in a swimming pool. If you try to hold the beach ball under the water, that requires a lot of energy. Your arms tremble from the effort. Your attention is taken completely by the need to keep the ball underwater and you hardly notice anything else around you. The ball must and will stay under the water. Eventually, you realise it isn't possible to continue; the buoyancy of the beach ball will always win. Suddenly, the ball will shoot out of the water and then drift gently away on the surface. This is how it works with feelings. Pushing your feelings down like the beach ball, whether consciously or not, requires energy. The harder you need to push to keep those emotions and memories underwater (out of your conscious mind), the less energy you have left for other things – and for everyday life. Feelings need to be felt.

You've got to feel it, to heal it.

If you use all your power to push down or push away your negative feelings, you also risk pushing away all your feelings, even the positive ones. Some women describe this as being unable to feel anymore, just emptiness.

"I was terrified during the journey from my house to the hospital. I had wanted to give birth at home and everything was going well until the pushing stage, which didn't work. The midwife said we had to go to the hospital. I assumed an ambulance would take me, but she said cheerfully: *"Your baby hasn't come out after an hour of pushing; he's not going to fall out during the drive to the hospital."* She said she would drive behind us. If there was a problem we were to stop by the side of the road. The road was very busy and I was very frightened. My husband was unaware of my fear, he was completely focused on getting us safely to hospital. The midwife told me not to put the back rest of my seat back as that might allow the baby to come out. Sitting upright made me feel like I was sitting on my baby's head. I barely dared to breathe and was unable to puff through my contractions. For me this was the worst part of the birth. It felt like a never-ending film in slow motion. Our baby was born an hour after we arrived at the hospital. I can remember very little of that hour. When they laid her on my stomach after using the ventouse, my only thought was: take her away and clean her up. I felt no maternal instinct, no love. In the first weeks following the birth I felt very little emotion, as if I were under a glass dome. I did what I had to, nodded obligingly when everyone said how wonderful it was, but I couldn't feel anything. Just emptiness. I wasn't sad or depressed, just empty. My uterus was empty and I was empty. My head was empty too. I kept forgetting things and found it hard to concentrate when I went back to work. The concentration problems eventually led me to seek help. Once I had processed the birth experience – where the lowest point was the drive to the hospital – the feeling of emptiness vanished. I can now laugh and cry again instead of walking around like a zombie." (Rachida, 26 years old)

The three basic psychological needs

As I stated in the introduction, you are (unfortunately) not the only person for whom labour was far from perfect. Your negative thoughts and feelings resulting from the birth do not make you a whiner or an attention-seeker. They do not determine how good a mother you are or define your relationship with your baby. *"Yes, I have something wonderful from the experience"*, can be expressed together with *"No, that doesn't make it a positive experience"*.

Research shows that almost a quarter of women giving birth for the first time have unpleasant feelings about their experience three years later. For women having a second (or third, or fourth) child, that number is one in eight. And you thought you were the only one!

So, why do so many women have a negative view of their labour? In addition to the important basic needs such as food, clothing and shelter, all humans – including you – have three basic psychological needs:

1. To feel safe and valued
    ("I matter", "I belong");
2. To believe in their own ability and to be taken seriously
    ("I can do it", "I'm good enough", "I am respected", "I feel competent");
3. To be allowed to choose, to be responsible for their own decisions or to have the space to make their own decisions
    ("I decide for myself", "I am responsible", "I do what I want").

Hardly anybody is able to completely fulfil these three basic psychological needs, therefore we continue to challenge ourselves and to grow and develop.

When we go through harrowing experiences, at least one of these basic needs is unfulfilled. Often it is two, or even all three of them. Many women whom I have coached in processing their birth experience have said that they didn't feel safe during labour. The rapport with the medical professionals was unsatisfactory or they didn't feel as though they were being taken seriously because they had no say in the decisions taken by the doctors during the birth. Moreover, many women have a feeling of having failed during childbirth.

Core issues

An unpleasant birth is even more painful when it hits a core issue in your life. Core issues are like a common thread recurring through your life, each time in a different form, changing slightly depending on the situation. Core issues are also known as a negative/damaged self-image, a cognitive (thinking) error or a negative self-concept.

"The midwife asked if perhaps I was afraid to keep pushing. That made me feel like I was failing. I had been pushing like mad for an hour, how could she say I was afraid to push? Help me, if I'm not doing it right. Coach me. When I noticed that she didn't believe I could do it, I too lost my confidence: my courage literally sank into my legs. Later, in the medical report I read 'mediocre pushing technique'. It was like reading 'failed' on an exam paper." (Eva, 38 years old)

"He just cut me, without asking, and I still haven't forgiven him for it. That sound of cutting will stay with me forever. As soon as he had done it, the baby flopped out and everyone was happy – everyone except me. Friends told me later that their doctors had always warned them when they were about to perform an episiotomy, or asked their permission before doing it. I didn't hear my doctor ask me anything. He mumbled something incomprehensible and then I heard the scissors. I had written in my birth plan that I did not want 'any intervention without consultation'. I felt like a piece of meat, as if I didn't matter, as if I were just the packaging that needed to be removed to get to the baby. To them, the baby was important; I wasn't. I was assaulted when I was a teenager and this experience brought that memory back to me: as if I didn't matter..." (Monica, 30 years old)

"During labour I felt like a small child, although at that time I was a 38-year-old career woman. I'm a single mother (by choice) and during the birth I suddenly missed my own mother, who passed away when I was still a child, enormously. I clung to the nurse and the midwife. I even started addressing them in a formal, polite way, just as my mother had taught me, although I consciously hadn't used that sort of language in years. The midwife joked about it and said I didn't have to be so formal. I didn't find it funny at all. I felt like a helpless and powerless eight-year-old child and I wanted my dead mother to come and rescue me." (Marion, 41 years old)

"Only afterwards did I realise how unsafe I had felt when giving birth in the hospital. I sat crying silently under the shower, completely alone. My husband was watching football on the television in the labour room and every now and then, dutifully called over: *"Are you alright, darling?"* The midwife on call was not one I knew and I hadn't 'clicked' with her. It seemed to me that all the staff were busy watching football and were annoyed that I had gone into labour during the World Cup finals. I would have loved for my contractions to stop. That feeling of being alone reminded me of how alone I had felt during my parents' divorce. Back then, I had also cried silently in the shower because I didn't want to upset my parents with my own grief. It was hard enough for them to look after themselves and to deal with each other." (Debbie, 27 years old)

"I was given a shot of pethidine, to curb the pain and then found myself completely spaced out. They could have warned me about that, if I had known I would never have opted for it. It actually made me hallucinate – it was frightening. Even after the drug was supposed to have left my system, my head felt foggy. When anyone spoke to me it sounded like they were standing underwater. I couldn't understand what they were saying, what they meant, what they expected from me. The pethidine made me lose any control I may have had over my delivery, whereas it's very important to me to have control and power over my life. After I gave birth, being in control became a compulsion for me." (Veronica, 37 years old)

If one of your basic psychological needs is unmet in your life and that same need is not met while you are giving birth, it can cause added pain and sadness. Once again, you have the feeling that you don't belong, that you aren't good enough, that your limits and your opinion are not respected and that everything is decided for you without you having a say, that you are doing what others want you to do instead of what you want to do. This puts a negative smear on your birth experience and confirms – without you realising it – an earlier negative conclusion you had made about yourself. The more often you experience something that confirms your negative self-concept, the deeper the pattern becomes etched into your system, and the stronger your emotional response when the raw spot is touched.

A negative birth experience touches your deepest core because you must both literally and figuratively expose yourself when you birth your child. You absorb everything that is said and done, even though it may seem to your partner and the medical professionals that you have retreated into yourself.

Luckily, with time, most women are able to process distressing birth experiences. The following chapter tells you what you can do by yourself and how to recognise the signs that you may need outside help.

Renée's

STORY

I had enjoyed being a teacher for years. After the birth of our first child I managed to pick up relatively easily where I had left off. How different it was when our second child was born! Towards the end of my maternity leave, I had a terrible feeling about going back to work. I didn't feel ready. However, I went back as planned. I had always been a popular teacher – to the extent a teacher can be popular with teenagers. But after my maternity leave, I was unable to maintain order in the classroom. The week before I finally gave up, I had sent four pupils out of the classroom. I had an increasingly short fuse. Just one incident would make me explode. I also often lost my train of thought in the middle of explaining something. While the pupils were working on an assignment, I just stared into space. I tried to do as much as possible on auto-pilot. Yet, my auto-pilot was not functioning. Correcting papers became arduous. I had to read everything twice. Because of this, I found myself working in the evenings and during the weekends more and more often. I clung to my work, it was my anchor. But nightmares were preventing me from sleeping and I trembled with exhaustion when I faced the class. And still I carried on.

After a few meetings, the head of the school advised me to take temporary sick leave. The work doctor warned me I was heading for a burnout. That was the final blow. For months, I had been pushing harder and harder to keep up, crossing my own limits. Suddenly, I literally had to lie down and I found it impossible to get up again. My husband took time off work to look after us.

I couldn't even care for the baby, except to breastfeed; luckily, that still worked. I slept and I cried. I cried and I slept. This lasted for two weeks.

The GP prescribed medication, which helped me to calm down enough to leave my bed and look after the children. That was the most I could manage. A friend and fellow teacher lent me Diana's book. I recognised myself in a number of the anecdotes and began to see a link between my ultra-fast labour and my present condition. It had gone so quickly, I had barely had time to crawl out of the bath and gave birth to my child, on my hands and knees, next to the toilet. The midwife was just in time to catch the baby. She still had her coat on and her equipment bag was still in the bedroom. By the time the assistant arrived, I was already lying back in bed. My husband joked that the midwife could have arrived a few minutes later, that he could have delivered the baby. He joked with the assistant that she had an easy cleaning-up job – just a quick mop of the bathroom floor. How strange that I couldn't remember how I had climbed out of the bath, how I ended up on all fours on the bathroom floor and delivered my baby there. But his silly jokes – even now – I remember word for word.

I had prepared myself for a hospital birth and was completely taken by surprise by the home birth. I couldn't comprehend it. I smiled politely along with the visitors, but whenever I was alone I kept going over the birth in my head. I tried to accept that my body had done what it needed to do, without my head being able to keep up. I had always functioned the other way around: hard work, planning and perseverance; my head always took the lead to reach my goals. But now I could neither trust my head nor my body. The expectation that after ten weeks I should be back at work to pick up where I had left off as if nothing had happened defeated me. I couldn't get into the right mode for work. The shock of the delivery was still in my body, and it hijacked half of my head and all of my memory. I wasn't capable of functioning normally. After a few sessions with a coach, I was able to slowly start work again. I began with small tasks and gradually expanded my activities. With hindsight, I should have started work much more gradually, slowly building up to the full extent of the job.

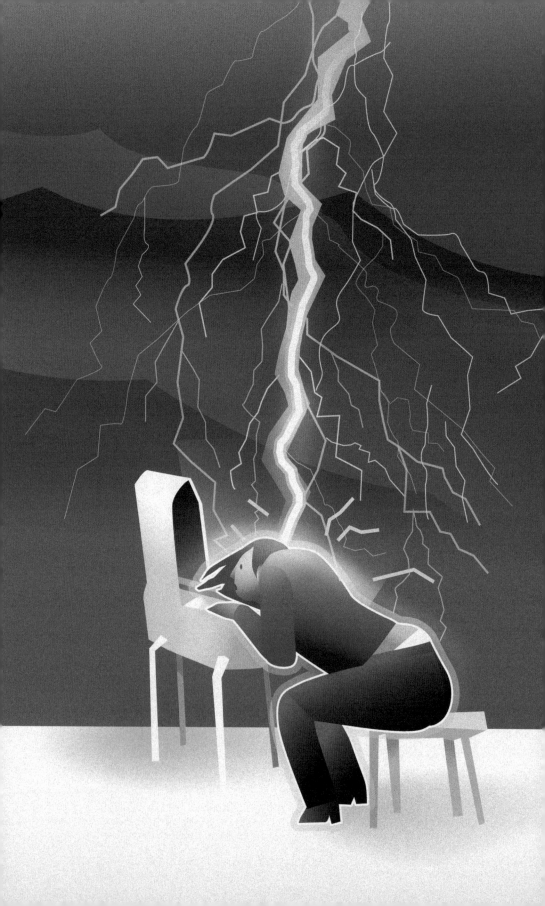

CHAPTER 2

Giving birth as a dividing or fracturing line; "before", "after" and a "different" person

Giving birth is an exceptional event that triggers exceptional emotions. These can be positive emotions, but also negative ones. For women who experience their labour as (very) disturbing, it is different again. These women might relate to the illustration on the opposite page, being "struck by lightning" during childbirth. During the birth they feel like "something" powerful has changed, making them feel different from the way they felt before. The birth represents a clear dividing line:

- "Before giving birth I was never anxious; after it, I was afraid of loud noises, afraid of the dark, afraid of losing people I loved."
- "Before giving birth I was always on top of things, I was eager to be a part of every adventure, every party. Since the birth I prefer to sit at home, as much as possible with the curtains closed. I do as little as possible, everything seems like too much. I avoid my friends. I can't even bear the thought of going to parties."
- "Before the birth I had never had nightmares or scary dreams; after the birth, I was tormented by them every night. I was afraid of going to sleep for fear of being woken by those terrible dreams."
- "Before the birth I rarely felt glum; since the birth I am pessimistic about everything, always expecting the worst to happen. I don't look forward to anything; everything has a dark shadow over it. I don't recognise myself anymore."
- "Before giving birth I enjoyed watching birth programmes on TV; since the birth I switch channels as soon as there is something to do with childbirth. I cannot even listen to my friends' birth stories – it makes me break out in a cold sweat."

- "Before the birth I was mostly unruffled, now I'm like a box of dynamite with a very short fuse. The smallest things can make me explode and my own fits of rage terrify me."
- "Before the birth I liked to plan things out; since the birth I have become a compulsive control freak, a sort of exaggerated version of my former self. I see myself doing it, I'm bothered by it, but I can't stop."
- "Before the birth I was an emotional person; since the birth I feel very little emotion, almost none, just emptiness."
- "Before giving birth I took things as they came, now I worry about what might happen, what might have happened, what I could have done or said differently, what others think of me. I worry constantly about the most random and trivial things. It's exhausting, but I can't seem to stop."

Partners/spouses can also be affected by a traumatic birth experience. The lightning can also have struck them during the experience, making them feel like a different person afterwards (see Chapter 5).

The normal way of processing a traumatic event

Your brain connects new experiences and influences with the information, knowledge, experience and memories it is has already stored. It tries to find the most suitable category to store this new information in a way that makes sense. To which category does this experience belong, where does it fit best? Your brain attempts to uphold the way you see yourself (self-image), other people (perception of others) and the world (world view), in order for these three perceptions to continue to "make sense".

During an intense experience such as childbirth, if something happens that doesn't feel right, or that feels threatening, your brain often doesn't have enough processing power to deal with it. Therefore, the images, thoughts and feelings become stored, "unprocessed", like a packing box that hasn't been unpacked yet.

Your brain saves this information to attend to at a later – calmer – stage. The brain rapidly stamps the event as "life-threatening" and switches to "survival mode". Survival mode gives you three options: *fight, flight or fright/freeze*. Escape (flight) is no option when giving birth. Fighting is possible to a limited extent. The third option is to freeze up and – seemingly resigned – to submit to what is happening to you. This is also referred to as *"tonic immobility"*: you are rigid with fear or paralysed from shock.

This can be frightening to go through, but it is actually a natural response for your brain to an abnormal or overwhelming event. In order to survive, the brain prioritises obeying urgent commands (such as to listen to the doctor and follow her instructions), above processing and integrating the information (what is actually happening to me right now and do I want it?). Once you, your brain and your body are back in a restful state, once you feel well and safe again, the memories (images, sounds, thoughts and feelings) resurface so they can be processed. If, at that moment (in the NOW), you feel secure, you can acknowledge these memories easily and process them in your own time.

Different people process intense experiences in different ways. This can be through a combination of the following:
- Talking about it;
- Collecting information, in order to have a complete view of what happened so you can understand why things happened the way they did;
- Writing down your story;
- Crying;
- Listening to music;
- Taking long walks in the countryside;
- Doing something creative;
- Gardening;
- Distracting your thoughts by playing computer games, reading, watching TV or films;
- Going back to work.

If you are able to process a distressing birth in the normal way, the painful images, memories and thoughts begin to fade over a few weeks and become less threatening. Your emotions are not as deep. At first, you think about the birth and want to talk about it very often. Slowly, this lessens and hours and days can go by without you thinking about it. You start to see your birth as a remarkable story, but it is a completed story. It happened as it happened. It's a shame, but too bad. You don't harbour any guilt. You were not able or willing to do it another way. It is fine as it is. It is "finished".

"It helped me to go for walks. I walked for hours through the woods every day with the buggy. I told everyone I was doing it in order to lose my pregnancy weight but it was mainly to lose the restlessness that I had felt inside since the birth. I had to go outside, even if it was raining. My son would lie in the buggy with the rain cover over him and I would stumble through the woods like a drowned rat in an awful raincoat. My husband and most of my friends worked full-time, I didn't have many people to meet up with on weekdays during my maternity leave, so I kept hiking through the woods, pushing the buggy. Often, tears ran down my cheeks. I kept walking until I felt peaceful inside. Only then would I head home. There was something very comforting in the woods. The walking really helped me avoid sinking into postnatal depression." (Naima, 24 years old)

"My homework was to start exercising again, because that was what had given me energy before I gave birth. I joined a group of mothers who exercised outdoors, coached by an instructor who was also a mother (and therefore not ultra-toned). It was a sort of boot camp for new mothers. That was incredibly good for me, every Saturday morning, no matter the weather, to leave my husband and child at home and pull the door shut behind me. Just for a while I didn't have anybody to be responsible for. As soon as I was on my bike I felt like my old self again. I am convinced that that one hour of outdoor exercise every Saturday helped me break the negative cycle I was in." (Manon, 37 years old)

"During my pregnancy I had decided to take parental leave straight after my maternity leave, allowing me to stay at home until the end of the year. That seemed like a wonderful idea... until my baby was born. I found I could not sit at home. That autumn it rained almost every day and I felt like the walls were closing in on me. All my friends were at work and I was bored senseless. I became more and more irritable. Eventually I decided to go back to work earlier than planned and to spread out my parental leave. Working helped me get back into my rhythm. It gave me satisfaction and this in turn lifted my mood. The fact that I was working made me appreciate much more the time I spent caring for my son on the days I was at home."
(Doris, 38 years old)

The normal way of processing a traumatic event – what you can do yourself

Many women have a feeling of having failed when they experience a traumatic birth. But how can you have failed when you have reached your goal? You were pregnant, with the goal of having a baby. Your child was born, therefore you reached your goal. If the circumstances or the position of the baby were unfavourable or your body did not produce enough labour hormones (oxytocin) or pain-reducing hormones (endorphins), that is not "failing" but "bothersome". This change in perspective makes a huge difference to your experience.
If you believe you have failed, you can feel responsible for the way your delivery went. If you think of it as a bother, it isn't your fault; it's just how the circumstances were. The checklist below is from Klaas Wijma's Traumatic Event Scale (TES-B) screening list to identify Postpartum Post-Traumatic Stress Disorder (PP-PTSD).

The following questions can help you identify to what extent your negative birth experience still affects your life today.

- Do you think about your birth in a negative way/with an unpleasant feeling?   yes / no
- During the birth did you ever feel that your life was in danger?   yes / no
- Were your physical or psychological boundaries crossed during the birth?   yes / no
- Did you feel during the birth that your baby's life was in danger?   yes / no
- Do the memories of the birth influence your (daily) activities in a negative way?   yes / no
- Do you have memory blanks for parts of your birth experience?   yes / no
- Do you notice that you have palpitations, sweating or other bodily reactions when you think about your birth experience?   yes / no

- Are you sometimes assailed by memories of the birth? yes / no
- Do you have nightmares or bad dreams about the birth? yes / no
- Do you sleep less well than before giving birth (without counting being kept awake by your baby)? yes / no
- Have you felt tired or lethargic since the birth? yes / no
- Do you think less well of yourself, other people or the world since the birth? yes / no
- Do you blame yourself for things that happened or did not happen during the birth? yes / no
- Do you feel shame or guilt with regard to the birth? yes / no
- Do you try not to talk or think about the birth? yes / no
- Do you try to avoid people or situations that remind you of the birth? yes / no
- Are you more irritable than before giving birth? yes / no
- Have you had memory or concentration problems since the birth? yes / no
- Are you more jumpy/on edge than before the birth? yes / no
- Do you have trouble getting excited about things you enjoyed doing or looked forward to before the birth? yes / no
- Do you feel responsible for the manner in which the birth played out? yes / no
- Do you suffer from intense feelings, thoughts or emotions that you didn't have before you gave birth? yes / no
- Is an earlier birth experience making you (more) anxious about the next one? yes / no

(Written) assignment

If the questions in the box above have an effect on you or if you answer "yes" to more than five questions, I advise you to write down your birth story. Focus on your thoughts and feelings during the birth, rather than on the facts. This exercise isn't about how your midwife or gynaecologist might have summarised it in her report, it's about how you experienced the birth.

So, instead of writing: *"The midwife arrived at 10 o'clock. I was two centimetres dilated so she left and said she would be back three hours later"*, you could write: *"When the midwife left and said she would be back in three hours, I began to panic. How on earth was I supposed to get through the three hours alone with my husband?! They were the longest three hours of my life. I felt completely abandoned."*

Writing down your story helps to put order in the chaos of your memories. You unpack and then repack your messy packing box as it were.

By writing away your thoughts and feelings you literally see your story from a distance. For some women, it's easier to write the story while looking at photos of the birth; other women don't want to or are unable to look at photos. See what feels right for you, what helps you to write your story. Next, read your story out loud, for example to your partner, mother, sister, friend, midwife, gynaecologist or GP. This is often a very emotional moment, which is mostly followed by a great feeling of relief.

"At the postnatal check the midwife realised that I hadn't yet processed the birth. She asked me to write down my experience of the birth and made a new appointment for a couple of weeks later. I was tempted to make up an excuse to call off the appointment but my husband wouldn't allow it. The evening before the appointment he almost had to force me to write down my story. He even started it for me.

Once I started writing I couldn't stop. It was very emotionally intense; I went through a whole box of tissues. I wrote late into the night through my tears. The story was barely legible, my pen flew over the paper and I had cramp in my hand from writing. I never read the story over. I was exhausted when it was finished. It was a relief, as if I had given birth over again.

The next day I gave my seven-page story to my midwife. She gave it straight back to me to read aloud. When I said I couldn't do that, she gave me a box of tissues and a glass of water and said I could take all the time I needed. I read and cried; the midwife listened. It must have lasted an hour. Afterwards I felt relieved and liberated as if I had literally handed over to the midwife the burden of my story. She said she would keep my story in my file in case I wanted it back. I have never felt the need to take it back." (Ayse, 23 years old)

When writing and talking aren't enough and the healing process stagnates

It takes time and energy to process a traumatic event. There is no standard time limit for it. Everyone processes painful events in their own way and in their own time. If you are tense, tired or stressed, you are hit extra hard by images, sounds, thoughts and feelings. If everyday influences have been impacting you more strongly since the birth, where can you be expected to find the energy to process the birth? Think about it: you're dealing with broken nights, getting used to a new routine, (feeding) problems, insecurities... and on top of that you are assailed by the painful memories of the birth.

Your brain might decide not to open this particular "packing box" just yet, but to put it away with a big red danger sticker on it. Because of this your brain stays extra alert and you keep scanning your environment for possible dangers that resemble the unpleasant birth experience.

You think and expect the worst and are constantly alert and on edge. Your senses are heightened, you are in a constant state of awareness, ready to up and run at any moment, salvaging whatever you can. You don't remember the event itself (the birth) in an objective or neutral way, but with a stress reaction and a negative conclusion about yourself (every woman can give birth normally, except me, so I'm a loser). This gives you the tendency to view other hurdles, such as nursing problems, through the same lens. (All women are able to breastfeed except me, so I'm a loser.) If your baby cries, you put it down to the distressing birth. Instead of thinking: "Oh, my baby is crying, perhaps she's hungry or has a dirty nappy", you think "everyone can comfort their child except me, so I'm a loser and a bad mother". These negative thoughts and negative conclusions about yourself push you deeper into the pit.

"I became completely focused on breastfeeding, to the point of obsession. In my eyes the birth had been unsuccessful. I felt I had failed while giving birth and therefore I wanted to do everything possible for the breastfeeding to succeed. In the first few weeks I was occupied 24/7 with nursing, expressing milk, feeding tubes and syringes. The breastfeeding had to be successful, to make up for the failed birth. Almost every day my mother advised me: *'Just give him a bottle and be done with it.'* It made me want to strangle her. Through my perseverance, the breastfeeding was eventually successful, and this made me proud. However, the way in which I achieved it – almost compulsively demanding so much of myself – I don't think was normal with hindsight." (Eva, 33 years old)

Eva's delivery was obviously not "unsuccessful". The way in which she gave birth was very different from what she had hoped. After the event, Eva concluded that the birth – as she had planned it – was unsuccessful and she made up her mind that she had failed. Her partner and the midwife both saw it very differently. But whatever they said, Eva stuck to her conclusion that the birth had been unsuccessful.

It is normal not to want to think back to your negative birth experience and to avoid everything related to childbirth. For example, you might decide not to go to the pregnancy yoga reunion or to avoid visiting friends who have just had babies. In the short term, your brain uses these techniques to protect you against stress. In the long term, however, avoidance actually generates more stress. Part of your brain is still desperately trying to keep that messy packing box (which is now also in the wrong place) closed. This maintains your feeling that you're in danger and you remain uptight.

Four to six weeks is a normal recovery period after an intense event, before you start to feel like yourself again, both physically and mentally. That's why the postnatal check is offered after six weeks. If you find that you have more questions about the delivery a few weeks or months later, make a new appointment to discuss them. It will help you to process the event if you get answers to your questions and you understand what happened. Your questions might include the following:

- What happened exactly and in what order?
- Which considerations did you make as a midwife or doctor? Which factors did you have to consider/weigh up?
- Why did you make certain decisions?
- Could it have been done differently?
- If you were in the same situation again would you make the same professional decisions?
- What did you think of my behaviour during the birth?

It's useful to put your questions down on paper beforehand as you might be so overwhelmed during the meeting by your memories of the birth that you might forget what you wanted to ask. What was exceptional or unclear for you may have been routine for the caregiver. Extra explanation can provide the missing pieces of the puzzle and help your healing process along.

Shame and guilt

You may have the feeling that you screamed the house down while giving birth, even if your partner tells you this didn't happen. If the midwife tells you that she didn't notice your behaviour to be out of the ordinary, this can spare you some feelings of shame and guilt. It can also be a relief if she agrees that you did scream, but that this was not exceptional behaviour during childbirth.

Many women worry about what others (in this case, the midwife or doctor) think of them. Talking openly about your feelings of guilt and shame make them lose their power. Guilt strengthens the perception that you have failed and that you did (or didn't do) something that makes you responsible for the way your labour went. This prevents you from processing the birth. If it can help you to process your birth experience it's a good idea to make an appointment as soon as possible with the person who coordinated your birth. If you would like to read more about the (unnecessary) impact of shame and guilt, I strongly recommend the books of Brené Brown (see Bibliography).

Me? Traumatised? Surely not!

The word "trauma" sounds (too) dramatic for many people when associated with giving birth. They describe birth as "difficult, long, intense or distressing" but "traumatic" seems to go too far. Those around the new mother might reinforce this idea by putting into perspective or playing down her experience by saying *"You will have forgotten about it soon enough, that's how it was for me." "But you have such a beautiful baby out of it all!"* and other such remarks (see Chapter 1).

As a result, many women don't feel comfortable talking about their negative experience for fear of sounding like they are complaining too much. Childbirth isn't supposed to be a walk in the park, all mothers have been through it and pain is just a part of it. In this way, they stifle their feelings with their rational thoughts.

Unfortunately, some people can be scornful when talking about traumatic childbirth experiences. *"Giving birth was traumatic? These women clearly haven't fought in a war! Now that is traumatic! How do you compare that to a birth that lasts at most 24 to 48 hours!"* Of course, you can't compare a birth trauma on the same level as a war trauma. Psychologists make a distinction between trauma with a small t and Trauma with a capital T. The word trauma is defined as *"a physical or psychological wound, caused by an accident, operation or intense life event"*.

A traumatic event is an event:
· Over which you had no/insufficient/a negative influence;
· Which you experienced as distressing;
· In which you were (completely) overwhelmed;
· Which negatively affects, and therefore burdens, your psyche (your thoughts and feelings).

According to the DSM-5 (*Diagnostic and Statistical Manual of Mental Disorders*, which is used to diagnose and categorise psychiatric complaints), a Trauma (capital T) can come about following exposure to "an actual or threatened death, serious injury and/or sexual violence".

You can suffer trauma if you have personally been through a distressing event and also if you have been a witness to one (for example, if you saw your partner giving birth). Hearing the story of a loved one who has been through a distressing event can also make you traumatised yourself. Finally, certain professions (fire-fighters, police, medical professionals and soldiers) can also suffer trauma from disturbing events in the context of their work.
The chance that you have to deal with a disturbing or traumatic incident at some point in your life is around 60%. Sixty per cent! You are therefore more likely to be affected by a traumatic event than not.

For many women, a distressing childbirth experience is their first confrontation with trauma in their life. Childbirth-associated trauma is not always Trauma with a capital T, in the sense that your life was endangered or your physical integrity was threatened. But having your physical or psychological boundaries crossed at an extremely emotionally vulnerable moment in your life (during childbirth) can be traumatic (with a small t).

"Giving birth was one of the most distressing things I had ever been through. I wanted to forget the whole thing as quickly as possible and never have to talk about it again. I also had memory blanks of parts of the birth. I couldn't remember what had happened and that was fine by me. I focused on my child and picked my life back up as if the birth had not happened. When my daughter was nearly a year old, I started having nightmares about the birth. I didn't understand what was happening to me. Sometimes I was even assailed during the day by flashbacks of the birth – it was driving me mad. After her first birthday it became harder and harder for me to keep thoughts of the birth out of my head. New painful images would surface every time. This all made me feel down and nervous and I began to have trouble going to sleep, for fear of nightmares. When I asked my GP for sleeping pills he advised me to speak to a therapist about my birth experience. Of course, that was what I wanted to avoid, but the doctor didn't want to give me sleeping pills unless I first tried talking about it with someone. Eventually, I am glad he was so insistent. Within six weeks I felt much better and could sleep without pills again."
(Fiona, 29 years old)

Luckily, the majority of women are able to process their distressing birth experience within four to six weeks. They do this by talking about it a lot, writing down their birth story, crying and focusing on positive things, like their baby. Other women require professional help to let go of their experience, even if they tried exactly the same methods. This doesn't mean that the latter group of women can't do what the former group can do. You are not "weak" if you have experienced giving birth as traumatic. In these cases your brain and your body have simply stored the experience differently, making it much harder to process. Some (highly sensitive) women experience things more intensely than other women, whereby distressing events impact them more strongly and are stored differently in their brain.

A traumatic event is something that happens to you, not something you choose

It is important to understand that you can't help the fact that you have experienced giving birth as traumatic. For example, two people might witness the same car accident. For one of them it will be a traumatic experience; they will have nightmares, think about it all the time and afterwards will feel anxious and unsafe when driving. The other person might heave a deep sigh, tell the story to a few people and then never think of it again. With giving birth, it can be the same. Two women might have a comparable birth, but one will experience it as traumatic, while the other will find it unpleasant but won't suffer any negative consequences. The same is true for witnesses to an accident, catastrophe or birth. Even as a partner, mother or friend, you don't get to choose whether a distressing event is stored as a "traumatic" experience in your brain. It happens to you.

event

thoughts   feelings

If you picture the distressing event as a film, there is often one scene that is the most painful to look at. You can stop the film at that scene. Usually you would have linked a negative thought about yourself to that image, such as "I'm a bad mother" or "I'm doing it wrong, I'm failing", along with the corresponding negative emotions such as regret, guilt, fear (of death), hopelessness or helplessness. In this way, the event, together with its negative thoughts and feelings, is stored in your brain as a danger triangle, written into your hard drive. If you don't do anything about this, your risk of suffering depression or anxiety is almost three times higher.

A distressing birth can bring back memories of earlier negative experiences, such as sexual abuse, a serious accident you were involved in or (the fear of) losing someone you love. In some cases, it isn't just one incident that causes the symptoms but an accumulation of experiences.

"At the start of labour, during an internal examination, the gynaecologist gave me a membrane sweep. He didn't explain exactly what he was doing while he did it; he just said he was going to help me a bit to get the contractions going properly. To me it felt like he was moving very roughly inside me, as if he was using his fist to pull my uterus down. I was completely overcome by this and was incapable of saying anything. I already had the feeling my words were getting stuck in my throat as if my throat was being held closed. That feeling came back again during a coaching session to talk about my birth experience. The coach asked if the gynaecologist had overstepped my boundaries when he – unexpectedly for me – performed the sweep. When I confirmed this, she asked whether I had ever had that feeling before. Immediately, memories of my first boyfriend flooded in. He had been very rough with me and had pushed me into going much further sexually than I was prepared for then, at the age of 14. Because I was so in love with him, I didn't protest. Not to him, or anyone else, even though until then I had always been able to speak to my mother about everything. The memory was so powerful, it made me feel like that 14-year-old girl again. I felt again how alone I had been at that moment because I didn't dare tell my mother about it.

My boyfriend maintained that this was normal, that it was what couples did when they were in love. I hadn't thought about that painful memory for years. In the meantime I had been with a man for 15 years who did respect my boundaries sexually. It was strange how the two unpleasant experiences were apparently interwoven in my mind. It felt good to be able to process them both during the coaching session." (Josie, 36 years old)

What makes a traumatic birth experience different from other traumatic experiences?

A childbirth trauma is an exceptional type of trauma, different from all other types of trauma. Giving birth is, for many women, one of the most intense events of her life in any case. It is an event women recall regularly, when their child has a birthday. This is why it is good to have pleasant (or at least neutral) sentiments about the birth of your child. Every mother wishes for her child to have the best possible start in life (outside of the womb). A traumatic birth may fall into the trauma with a small t according to the strict DSM-5 definition, but for many women it's a double trauma, because it occurs in such an important and notable moment in their lives. If you are in a car accident on a random day in your life it can be traumatic. If you have a car accident on your wedding day, that can be extra traumatic. Not only do you need to process the pain of the accident but a beautiful event (your wedding day) will always be tainted by it. To draw a parallel with giving birth, a traumatic birth experience might give you the feeling that "one of the most beautiful moments of your life" has been taken away from you. It is also extra burdensome to have to process a traumatic event in a period that already demands a lot of adjustment in your brain. You need to fit the arrival of the baby in your life, adapt your life to the baby, manage your pregnancy hormones, recover physically, etc. This is why you might experience a traumatic birth as a double trauma (with a small t).

Traumas you have suffered from accidents, wars and attacks are painful by definition. They are painful from start to finish. In contrast, giving birth usually starts off pleasantly. As new parents you generally look forward to the arrival of your baby. You've prepared yourselves well for the birth, perhaps followed a birth preparation course, doing pregnancy yoga or making a birth plan together. These things make it seem like the birth can be planned. This is an illusion! But this illusion creates the impression that the trauma could have been prevented, if you had been better prepared or if you had really done your best. This is nonsense. A trauma is something that happens to you, you cannot prepare yourself for it, just as you cannot prepare yourself for an accident. It's even worse when a "pleasant" birth suddenly becomes a very distressing event.

The midwife or gynaecologist, whom you thought seemed so nice, is decidedly less nice during the birth. You feel abandoned by her/him, you feel that your boundaries are being overstepped, that they are not listening to you, that you have not received enough information or explanation, or are not being taken seriously. The practitioner whom you had hoped and expected would support, coach and guide you, seems to you to have turned into a kind of abuser during the birth.

You may feel unsafe during the birth and worry about your or your baby's health, but you can do very little to bring yourself and your baby to safety. You may feel like you have surrendered to the midwife or doctor in charge of your birth. They are doing their best to make you feel safe and to monitor and promote your health, but in spite of this you can feel unsafe. Even if the doctor says that your and your child's life are not in danger, you may still believe they are.

During childbirth there is no way back. You might feel that you have been left to your fate. There is no escape. For some traumas, you can avoid repeating the trauma (for example, you can decide to not drive anymore, quit the army, or work in the office rather than behind the counter at a bank), but you cannot do this with childbirth once you are pregnant again or if you would like to have another baby. You also cannot avoid the "product" of the trauma – the baby. On the contrary, you are expected to cherish this "living reminder of your trauma" because your baby is completely dependent on you.

Childbirth can affect your sex life. After delivery your genital area might be painful due to a cut, tear, stitches or haemorrhoids. You and your partner might also experience your genitals differently after you have given birth. Unfortunately, a traumatic birth experience often has a negative impact on your sex life. Your genitals might keep reminding you and your partner of the delivery, with many negative physical, psychological and relational consequences (see Chapter 5). Some women are afraid to undergo a cervical smear after giving birth because they don't want to have their feet in stirrups again. Avoiding gynaecological tests and cervical smears can have consequences for your health.

Trauma can lead to Post-Traumatic Stress Disorder (PTSD)

As we have seen, almost a quarter of women who gave birth to their first child (and one in eight women in the case of a second or subsequent child), remember the birth in a negative way three years after it took place. In 1–3% of cases, women are diagnosed with Post-Traumatic Stress Disorder (PTSD). Increasingly, the correct term PP-PTSD is used: Postpartum Post-Traumatic Stress Disorder. For the sake of simplicity I have chosen to use the acronym PTSD in this book.

Psychological complaints following childbirth are often not recognised as symptoms of PTSD, because most medical professionals do not yet know enough about this specific subject. Postpartum depression (PPD, also known as postnatal depression) is sometimes incorrectly diagnosed and treated, because doctors and midwives do not recognise the symptoms as symptoms of PTSD. In these cases, the result (PPD) is treated instead of the cause (PTSD complaints resulting from a traumatic birth experience). Unfortunately, only a fraction of women dare to bring up their complaints with their doctor. The sense of shame is often too great, because the baby is healthy.

Women believe they shouldn't keep complaining about their birth experience because it happened so many months or years ago. Many women bury – consciously or not – the painful memories of the birth. This works to some extent for some women, until they are pregnant again and giving birth again becomes unavoidable. A number of women decide against a new pregnancy in order to avoid having to go through the (birth) trauma again. Partners may also be traumatised by the birth and therefore not want to go for another pregnancy (see Chapter 5). Therefore a traumatic birth experience can have consequences for the size and make-up of your family. In many cases, there is partial or *subthreshold* PTSD. This means that women suffer from some, but not all of, the symptoms listed in the following paragraph. Because of this, the PTSD diagnosis is not established and these women are not included in the statistics. Unfortunately, the vast majority of women with psychological complaints resulting from childbirth do not seek help and suffer in silence. That is the purpose of this book: to help you get relief from your symptoms.

Finally, PTSD is often not diagnosed because women only seek help much later – months or even years after the event. This happens, for example, when they have trouble at work due to tension or a burnout, if they suffer from depression or anxiety and are then treated for these complaints, while in essence they are suffering from untreated PTSD, which causes the other mental issues. I estimate therefore that the actual number of women suffering from their upsetting birth experience is much higher. I suspect we are only seeing the tip of the iceberg.

Symptoms of Post-Traumatic Stress Disorder (PTSD)

If you have been suffering for more than four weeks after an intense, shocking or traumatic event from complaints such as (1) reliving the event, (2) avoidance, (3) negative thoughts and moods, and (4) heightened awareness, and this is affecting your everyday life in a negative way, you might have PTSD. The way in which you react doesn't help you to process the distressing event. Instead of gradually getting better you begin to feel worse.

1. Reliving the event

It's normal to relive the event in the first weeks after giving birth. You process what you went through piece by piece. If after four weeks, the birth still feels "unfinished" and you still find yourself "redoing" parts of the birth, this could be a sign of PTSD. You are unexpectedly assailed by memories of the birth (also called flashbacks or intrusions). The corresponding feelings can be just as potent as during the birth. You might be overwhelmed by sounds, smells, images, physical reactions, thoughts and feelings. This can happen, for example, when you hear someone else tell their birth story or if you think of a friend who is due to give birth in the near future.

Going back to the hospital where you gave birth, even if it's to a completely different ward or to visit a sick friend or family member – you might suddenly be violently reminded of your birth experience. This can also occur for no apparent reason. Many women suffer from very upsetting or frightening dreams about their birth experience.

Reliving the painful event is one thing. The meaning you give to the reliving and memory, the label you attach to it, determines how badly you are suffering from the memories. Some women tell me tearfully that they thought they were going mad because they were regularly assaulted by flashbacks. It might be a relief for you to know that flashbacks are a symptom of PTSD.

"I had had a disturbing birth, but a beautiful child, and life went on. After a couple of months I went back to the gynaecologist to have an IUD fitted. As I walked into the hospital I broke out in a sweat. It was a warm day so I didn't pay too much attention to that. Sitting in the waiting room, I had another sweat attack. I also felt stifled.

I thought I was going to faint. I told the receptionist I needed to make a phone call and went out. Once outside, I sat on a bench with my back to the hospital. This helped me calm down slowly. When I went back to the gynaecology unit I felt dizzy and claustrophobic again. I tried breathing very gently into my stomach, which, luckily, made the panicky feeling disappear. When I lay on the examination table with my feet in the stirrups, it suddenly felt like I was giving birth again. I wanted to scream but no sound came out. The gynaecologist had already inserted the speculum. She was about to put the coil in when I jumped off the table because I needed to throw up. She referred me to a coach to help me process the birth." (Eve, 40 years old)

2. Avoidance

It's normal to try to avoid thinking about a disturbing event, in this case, your birth experience. In the short term this can help, but furiously repressing memories takes up a lot of energy in the long run. You would be better off using that energy for the healing process. When you ignore your memories out of fear, you are just giving them extra weight. Avoiding them makes them "heavier"; the danger triangle becomes larger and you become more anxious.

This brings you into a negative spiral of fear and avoidance that feeds itself, leading you to:
- not want to see (any more) photos of the birth;
- not want to talk about it;
- not want to hear other people's birth stories;
- avoid visiting new mums and their babies;
- never want to get pregnant again because you never want to give birth again;
- insist on delivering the next baby by C-section, because you're afraid of a vaginal birth;

- want to deliver your next baby by yourself because you don't trust midwives or gynaecologists anymore;
- avoid or delay gynaecological examinations and cervical smears, which could impact your health.

"I nearly bled to death when I gave birth and had a miscarriage after that where I also lost a lot of blood. During the miscarriage I had to be lifted out of my house by the fire brigade as I couldn't walk down the stairs because of the blood loss. The neighbours were watching, which I found mortifying.

Nobody could give me a guarantee that it wouldn't happen again the next time, so I didn't want to risk another pregnancy. I also didn't want to talk about the first birth or the miscarriage and avoided anything that had to do with childbirth. I didn't visit my friends when they had just given birth. I pretended I didn't want to bother them with a visit at such a busy time, and instead I took them out for coffee and cake once they were back on their feet. A year later my husband wanted another child. I found it impossible to even discuss the issue and this led to a crisis in our relationship, which took us to see a coach. That was where I first heard about PTSD and began to understand what was happening to me." (Flora, 32 years old)

3. Negative thoughts and moods

Since the birth you have less pleasure in doing things. You don't enjoy your hobbies, socialising or exercise, while you were always enthusiastic about these things before the baby. You don't look forward to fun activities. You find those activities and the people you do them with (family and friends) much less appealing than before. It's as if you can't warm up to anyone or anything anymore.

You feel more down than you are used to, as if you are simply unable to be happy and positive anymore. Women describe this feeling as sitting under a glass dome, as if there is a filter over everything or as if there is a dark cloud on everyday things. You think badly about yourself, other people and the world in general ("I can't trust anything/anybody", "nobody cares how I feel") and you assume the worst, the most negative (doom) scenario. You also cannot remember parts of your birth experience.

"I felt like hitting the people who told me: *'But you got something wonderful out of it, didn't you?'* I didn't find my baby wonderful at all, or even nice. I wouldn't have cared if the whole motherhood thing had been taken away from me. I was on the point of calling work to ask if I could come back earlier from maternity leave, but didn't do it because I was afraid of their reaction, that they would think I was a bad mother. I was relieved to be able to go back to work when my leave was over, so it was extremely frustrating when I was unable to work to my usual standards because of concentration problems. My job had always been the most important thing to me. I felt more and more down. I was afraid I was sinking into postnatal depression. The coach asked if I thought there was a link with my harrowing birth experience and I immediately felt she had hit the nail on the head. The birth had indeed marked the start to all my problems." (Marie, 28 years old)

4. Heightened awareness (*arousal* or hyperactivity)

If you suffer from PTSD you can easily become over-sensitive. Any small stimulus can make you explode. You are much angrier, on edge and more emotional than before the birth. Unusual violent fits of rage are normal for women with PTSD following an intense childbirth experience. Those around you often put these outbursts down to "hormones", but you know that they aren't normal reactions because you don't have control over yourself in those moments. Women often shock themselves with their own negative reactions, thoughts and feelings. This in turn leads to feelings of guilt and shame. You don't feel able to relax anymore, or even to sit still. You have trouble remembering things and concentrating. You don't sleep well, are (over) tired and therefore more irritable. You are (over) protective of your baby, like a mother hen. You are continuously (hyper) alert, ready to fight or flee. It's tiring enough to read about these symptoms, let alone to have to live with them on a daily basis.

"Since the birth, loud noises and people hugging me unexpectedly from behind made me jump. I was over-protective of my daughter. With every sound she made, I rushed over to check on her, with every whimper I lifted her out of her cot. This disturbed her sleep patterns and mine too. I was very tired and at the same time in a state of high alert. My husband and my mother said I was making my daughter agitated, because I kept taking her out of her bed. I couldn't see that I wasn't giving her the chance to fall asleep by herself. Because I was so tired I was very irritable. My husband had to pay the price for this. At first he made jokes about it: *'Are those hormones bothering you again, honey?',* but after a few months he asked: *'When am I going to get my sweetheart back?'* I realised too that I wasn't myself anymore but had no idea why that was and what I could do about it. Only much later did I find out that I had been in shock because I had to have an operation to have my placenta removed, and that shock was still in my system a year later." (Frederique, 35 years old)

> PTSD is diagnosed if these four symptoms – reliving the event, avoidance, feeling low and heightened awareness – are present several times a week or every day, while the event itself (the birth) took place at least a month before. The symptoms negatively impact your daily life (yourself, your family, your relationship, your work, your social contacts). You are unable to resume your life as you were used to before the birth. Your symptoms are likely to have been triggered by the birth (because you didn't have them before giving birth). The following words are used by women to describe a distressing birth experience: helplessness, guilt, the feeling of having failed, panic, hell, fear of dying, fear the baby will die, lack of faith in the medical staff, disappointment in your partner, disgust, horror, revulsion at the baby, too much pain (I'm going to collapse), loneliness, sadness, the feeling of having been assaulted or raped. Chapter 3 further describes PTSD complaints that you can develop as a result of a traumatic birth experience.

Sophie's

STORY

Following a distressing miscarriage and curettage I became pregnant for the second time. This second pregnancy went perfectly. I felt fantastic and full of energy. However I didn't see how I would be able to hold down my fulltime job with a child and surprised everyone by handing in my resignation. I was sure about my decision; I knew it would be alright. And it was alright: once our eldest child was born I began working part-time in my husband's family business.

On one hand, I was not looking forward to giving birth. Such an unknown and uncontrollable event was not welcome to the control freak that I was. On the other hand, I approached it very practically. The child had to come out, anyone can give birth, I'm fit, so... bring it on! I went into labour in the evening. The contractions built up very slowly. By the following afternoon I couldn't stand the pain anymore. The doctor broke my waters in the hope that it would speed up the labour. At 6.30 in the evening I was given an epidural and an hour later I was fully dilated – but I had no urge to push, not even after an hour. I did push anyway but didn't know which way to do it. In total I pushed for about two and a half hours interspersed with breaks in which I had to puff. In the final half hour I was given medication through a drip to strengthen my contractions. My daughter's heartbeat had slowed almost to a stop. I could hear her little heart beating slower and slower. I thought of the little pink jacket I had bought her and was afraid she might never get to wear it. The tension within the medical team was palpable. What would be quicker: the ventouse or a C-section? The operating room team had already been called. The doctor looked at me and said: *"Now or never."* Three pulls with the ventouse and a hefty cut later, Catoo was born. Her Apgar score was two and she needed to be given oxygen in another room. My husband and I waited tensely. Luckily Catoo recovered within ten minutes.

I didn't remember anything of my first meeting with Catoo, although I had been looking forward to it so much. I was completely exhausted, had given everything and actually had a sort of blackout. I had missed the most precious moment of my life! The nurse wanted to help me breastfeed. Catoo was clearly ready for it but I wasn't yet. I felt a looming sense of responsibility. I was a mother now, and was expected to do everything I could in the interest of my child. That included breastfeeding her, even though I hadn't quite "landed" yet from the delivery. I obediently did what I was told. Catoo was doing well but things were not going well with me. My episiotomy wound got infected, breastfeeding didn't work and I had an over-enthusiastic nurse who told me ten times a day that I *"must enjoy it"*. I tried to keep visitors to a minimum, which was very unlike me. I felt more and more miserable. I told the professionals every day that I didn't feel well, but they assured me it was normal. I should have listened to myself properly. After a couple of days I was so sick that it became obvious this was not normal. I ended up in the hospital with a uterine infection. It may sound odd but this lifted a weight off my shoulders. For one thing, I was not imagining it; for another, I felt myself getting better from the antibiotics drip.

A year later I had recovered physically, but I found it hard to enjoy Catoo and my life as a mother. I had lost myself. I missed the energetic and cheerful Sophie that I had always been. I sometimes resented Catoo for changing my life so much. I constantly had the feeling of having to do things. Planning everything and carrying out what I had planned became my daily objectives. I was very hard on myself. I didn't feel depressed but was not really happy either.

Just before I fell pregnant again (a desired pregnancy, but faster than I had planned), I had hurt my back and got strong painkillers and muscle-relaxing medication from the doctor. I found out later that I should never have been given that medication in early pregnancy. I started having hefty stomach cramps and was afraid I was going to lose my child. For the remainder of my pregnancy I was worried I had endangered my baby's health.

My labour began well; the first internal exam showed I was already six centimetres dilated. But after that it went less quickly. For Kevin I also had to push for an hour, and his heartbeat also slowed dangerously. The gynaecologist decided to perform a C-section. They gave me medication to slow the contractions because I couldn't be admitted to the operating room straight away. When the gynaecologist left the room, the midwife told me to *"give it all I had"* and *"push as if my life depended on it"*. That felt so contradictory: whom was I to listen to? Whose "command" was I to obey? To push as if my life depended on it, or stop pushing and puff instead because the life of my child depended on that? When I was finally admitted to the operating room they made a final attempt to deliver Kevin with forceps, but he was positioned too high up for that. The C-section and recovery from it were harder than I had expected. Kevin was healthy but again, I wasn't doing so well. Once more I allowed the people who should have known better to convince me it was normal. A week later I was back in the hospital, again with a uterine infection. Once again I had a stressful period just after the birth. Once again I was focused on myself, my illness and my recovery and had no time to get used to Kevin.

I finally asked for help, but only a year and a half after Kevin was born. For three years I had had less energy, less enjoyment in things and neglected my physical condition. I processed my first birth experience with the help of EMDR (see Chapter 7). All kinds of emotions I had had during the birth resurfaced: agitation, anxiety, insecurity, doubt, helplessness, exhaustion, pain, lack of trust, despair, hopelessness, worry, fear that Catoo would not make it and relief when she was okay. Suddenly a mental image came back to me of my husband proudly carrying her back from the room where she had been given oxygen. I had completely forgotten that look in his eyes. It was the same with the sight of Catoo lying in my arms. It made me cry but this time they were tears of joy. So I had felt love for Catoo straight away. That feeling had escaped me in all the confusion that had followed her birth. In the days following the EMDR treatment, I noticed that Catoo came to sit on my lap or lie next to me more often, whereas she hadn't been such a cuddling type before then. My husband noticed it too. The feeling of unrest that I had been carrying inside for three and a half years slowly started slipping away. Catoo was a fussy eater and was treated for this by a specialized paediatrician. I found out that eating problems occur more often in children who experience a difficult birth. Catoo had EMDR therapy for this too in the hospital. She improved by leaps and bounds thanks to her therapy, and to mine. Our bond grew stronger; we understood each other better.

While out shopping one day, I came across a stone with the inscription "welcome, dear little girl". I bought it as a reminder of that period. I realised that I had bundled both my birth experiences into one box, slammed the door and thrown away the key. I had done that consciously, in order to keep myself going. But, in doing it, I had also thrown away a part of myself. I had stopped listening to my inner voice, and didn't dare trust myself anymore. This made me lose my compass and I was lost on all fronts. I listened and did what I was told by others instead of deciding my own way.

Hospital tests revealed that I had just 60% of my lung capacity. My coach remarked that I had been forcing myself to perform at 120% of my capability on just 60% of my battery charge. I made a plan to perform at 50% for home and work activities together so that I would have 10% capacity left over. My husband was a role model for me in this. I learned from him to let go and to delegate. Slowly, the old energetic Sophie began to reappear.

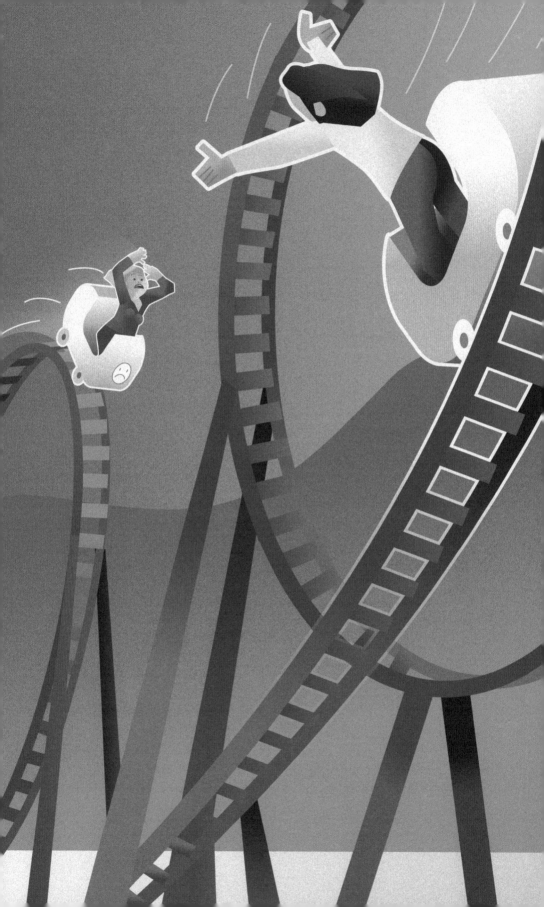

CHAPTER 3

A distressing birth
– how it affects you

A distressing birth experience brings about various physical and psychological complaints, which can range from mild to severe. In my practice I have noticed that women (and those around them) often don't make the connection between the distressing birth and the complaints/symptoms that develop, sometimes months, later. GPs, midwives and gynaecologists do not see the link either. Of course, not every psychological complaint is a consequence of the birth, but in my opinion, it isn't sufficiently explored whether the birth has played a role in the onset of psychological problems. In this chapter we will discuss the consequences of sleeplessness, worry, concentration problems, insecurity and the compulsive need for control, anxiety, depression, burnout and sexual abuse. At the end of the chapter there are a number of practical tips and exercises.

There is something missing

It is significant that women who experienced giving birth as traumatic often use words ending with "less", almost as a signboard; "there is something missing". The birth is the cause, the "something missing" (powerlessness, helplessness, desperation, hopelessness) is the result.

When you think about your birth experience do these terms feel familiar?
Powerless, helpless, pointless, desperate, useless, hopeless, worthless, indecisive, lack of respect, speechless, listless, out of control, ruthless, unable to be comforted, unfeeling, endless, merciless, senseless, heartless, lifeless, dispirited, restless, unloving.

"My son Kian was born much too early, at 34 weeks. I was still at work when my waters suddenly broke. In the hospital they tried to slow the contractions. They explained that the baby's lungs were not developed enough and therefore I was given medication through a drip. I had complete faith in the doctors' ability to stall my labour and tried to ignore the increasing stomach cramps I was experiencing. This turned out to be in vain, because an hour and a half later, Kian was born. I only needed to push a few times. I didn't know what was happening to me. The paediatrician took him straight away to another room and my partner went with them.

I lay stoically on the bed while the gynaecologist stitched me up. Somehow I didn't feel any panic. I felt nothing, but a sort of 'blankness'. I had expected to cry from happiness or something, but instead I just thought, *'Okay, the baby's here.'* Just like I was stating a fact, rather than feeling an overpowering emotion. I understood from the coaching sessions that I had gone into a 'freeze mode' during the birth; I simply took it in, as if I were frozen. While Kian was doing well, given the circumstances, I spent the first two weeks crying. Upon waking up I thought I was still pregnant. When I looked at him I didn't feel anything. Once Kian was allowed home he cried often and for great lengths of time. I didn't have a moment to myself. I can hardly remember anything from the first three months – I was purely in survival mode.

When asked: *'Do you feel like you were under attack, rather than giving birth?'* it seemed they had hit the nail on the head. Until I went into labour, my whole life had gone as I had expected and planned. Everything was under control. This was the first real setback I had had in my life. My sister gave birth to her first child without a problem and the time following the birth also went relatively smoothly. Why had everything been normal for her and so different for me? This gave me the feeling that I had failed.

The coach said: *'It sounds like you and Kian are both in shock from being under attack and, as with any attack, you need to give yourself time to process it. Try to have some compassion for yourself and for your son, as if you were listening to a friend's story.'* Under attack instead of giving birth – the realisation of what I had been through made me very emotional. Of course people needed time to recover

from an attack. That included babies. In the following sessions we discussed my sadness but also my anger that it had happened in that way. I felt robbed of my maternity leave. Instead of having some restful time off I was very busy looking after Kian. I resented him for that. One of the exercises I did taught me to direct my anger towards nature, towards what happened to Kian and me. Perhaps Kian cried so much because he hadn't been ready to be born. His plans were also disrupted by the early labour. I felt something change inside me. Now we could be angry together. The blame lay with nature, not with Kian or me. We had been under attack together by the premature birth."
(Ina, 35 years old)

In balance, or finding a balance

There are very few women for whom the birth and the ensuing recovery period goes exactly as they expect. There is a reason why they say you are pregnant for nine months and you "recuperate from your pregnancy" for another nine. After the arrival of every new family member it takes a while before you find your new balance. Moreover, the length of this period varies for each person, and depends on a number of variables. The more life events you go through in a short time the more you step out of balance. Some examples of positive life events are marriage, pregnancy, giving birth, renovating or moving house, but there are also negative events such as illness, loss of a loved one (such as your baby), involvement in an accident, serious illness, a (natural) disaster, miscarriage, job loss or financial worries. Life events – even the positive ones – temporarily upset your balance.

If you undergo more than three life events in one year you actually have twice as much chance of suffering physical or psychological complaints in that year.

Almost nobody is always "in balance". It's more realistic to learn to balance, like rope-dancers. They continuously correct their position, rocking from left to right while walking on the tightrope. Rope-dancers use a tool (a long stick or waving arms) to stay balanced. Who or what can help you to learn how to balance in this new phase of your life? The exercises at the end of this chapter will give you some guidance.

"On the questionnaire that I had to complete in preparation for the coaching session, I wrote that my objective for the therapy was *'to get back my old life, body and fun'*. The coach noticed that sentence immediately: *'You're setting yourself an impossible goal. Your life after having a baby can't be compared to your life before you became a mother. Pregnancy and motherhood change the bodies and the lives of most women. Yearning for what doesn't exist anymore won't help you. On the contrary, whatever you give attention to, grows, so as long as you keeping longing for a time that is now finished, you'll only end up further adrift.'* Later, when I sighed that I *'just wanted to be back in balance'*, she smiled and suggested: *'Shall we first look together at what you need to find your balance? Your life is upside-down at the moment, don't set the bar too high.'*

Just like that, a few words from that first meeting stayed with me and have proved to be a handle that I can hold on to on my road to recovery." (Lisa, 26 years old)

Take a closer look at your life

Take a moment to write down everything that has happened in your life this past year. All these events are stored somewhere in your head, but if you write them down, black on white, you have a much better overview.

Describe which life events, personality traits, physical changes and environmental factors might play a role:
• Has there been a change in your health status or fitness level due to your pregnancy and the birth?
• Which personality traits affect the way you deal with changes? (For example, are you a perfectionist or do you like to control what happens in your life?)
• Are there people in your circle who can offer practical or emotional support?
• Which emotionally intense life events have you been through in the last three years?

Clients often feel relieved when I fill in this template with them: *"It's actually quite a lot. I shouldn't be surprised that I feel the way I do."* If you can be understanding and charitable towards yourself, that is what I fervently wish for you. These exercises will hopefully replace the gnawing guilt with self-empathy. It's time to replace being hard on yourself with being gentle and kind to yourself. Being pregnant is tough, giving birth is hard, and it's not at all easy to look after a fully dependent baby who was delivered without an instruction manual. What a responsibility! It's probably also the first time in your life that you have someone around you 24/7. As you and your partner get to know your baby, and your baby gets to know you, you figure out the instructions together. After a while you know better than anyone that one type of cry means that the baby is hungry, another type means she needs to burp and still another means she needs a clean nappy. It's normal to need time to get used to each other. Don't expect too much from yourself.

"Never before in my life had I felt so accountable, so guilty and so useless as in my first months of motherhood. My mother and mother-in-law knew what my baby needed better than I did. If he cried, my mother would say: *"It sounds like he needs to burp."* Incredible! How could she possibly know that?

Before I knew it my mother had already picked him up, made him burp (how did she do that so fast?) and he was lying peacefully in her arms, looking up at her. I became increasingly miserable and was hardly able to get up off the couch. My mother and mother-in-law took over my son's care almost completely. The more they did, the more unsure of myself I became. In the first coaching session I made an overview of everything that had happened in my life over the past year: I had had a miscarriage, followed by an extra-worrying pregnancy with more blood loss, my father had had a (minor) brain haemorrhage, there had been a restructuring at my office, I had had a distressing birth experience, infected stitches, mastitis and a baby who cried a lot and had thrush in his mouth.

The coach asked me to look at the overview as if it were written about a friend. What would I say to that friend? I replied: *'I would put my arm around her and say: "This is impossible, sweetie, I'm not surprised you are overwhelmed, it's unbelievable how much you've been through this past year."'* The coach asked me to put my arms around myself and to say those words out loud to myself. It was a warm hug with warm, friendly words. It really helped!

In the months after that I regularly hugged myself and gave myself some words of encouragement, as if I were speaking to a friend. The coach also instructed me to take over the care of my son again as much as I could, in order to build up 'care miles' as she put it. In a notebook I recorded what I had done and how he reacted to me and this slowly built my confidence as a mother. She said I was writing an instruction manual for my child in that notebook, and that is indeed how it felt." (Elisa, 39 years old)

Bringing your weighing scales into balance: limiting the burden and strengthening the carrying capacity

As well as focusing on your life, it might help you to make an overview of your load and capacity.

In the first column, list the things that use energy (your energy drainers) and in the second, the things that give you energy (your energy providers/chargers). Alone, or with your partner or a friend or family member, think of how you can rebalance your scales. What changes do you need to make to limit the load and increase the carrying capacity? Can you delegate some tasks or ask people around you for help? What advice can you glean from friends with small children? Are the chores in your household fairly divided? The greater your load, the more important it is that your capacity matches up. Many people don't pay enough attention to this. They slump under their workload and this makes it even heavier. You can increase your capacity by looking after yourself well and recharging your battery (yourself). It might help to create a household chart with a division of tasks (see Chapter 5).

Often, women automatically take on extra tasks during their maternity leave because they're "not working anyway". In addition to this, women usually see things that need to be done in the house more than men do. This can lead to the division of tasks during the pregnancy being relatively balanced, namely 60% (woman) and 40% (man). During the weeks of maternity leave, before the arrival of the baby, it tends to shift without anyone noticing to 70% and 30% or even 80% and 20%. It's then very difficult to reverse that after the baby is born and once you are back at work.

Most new parents underestimate how many hours in the day they will be occupied with caring for the baby. It takes about eight hours a day: feeding the baby (eight to 12 times a day), washing the baby and changing nappies (five to eight times a day), burping the baby (during and after every feed), comforting, dressing and changing clothes (several times) – because the baby has dribbled/brought up milk or her nappy has overflowed – and doing extra laundry. This only refers to an average baby, not even one who cries more than others

"I got a shock when I filled in the household chart. Without realising, I had taken over almost all the household chores during my maternity leave. I was bored in the last weeks before the baby arrived and housekeeping, shopping and cooking gave me something to do. After our son was born we were both tired from the broken nights. I didn't want to burden my partner with getting up at night because he needed to go to work during the day and I was 'off'. After two months I was a complete mess. As soon as I saw on the chart everything I did (and everything my boyfriend didn't do) I got a shock. When I showed him the chart, he was shocked too. We made a new chart together that gave me breathing room and time to recover. From that point onwards, I make time to go outside walking every day instead of doing household chores. Two months on, my boyfriend found a cleaner through a colleague. He had always thought it was excessive to have professional help with household chores, but that was before we had a new daily task with the arrival of our son." (Fay, 30 years old)

Physical complaints

Most physical complaints stem from underlying physical causes. However, your body can also convey psychological problems through physical complaints. If you have been through trauma you can experience various physical symptoms, such as headaches, back pain, stomach ache, neck and shoulder pain and heart palpitations. As the saying goes: what the mind suppresses, the body expresses.

Let your doctor know if you experience physical complaints that you didn't have before giving birth. Thyroid problems, for example, can cause anxiety or depression. Deficiency of various nutrients, such as iron (low haemoglobin/Hb), vitamin B, vitamin D3 or omega-3 (DHA) can lead to physical illness as well as feelings of depression. While you are pregnant your baby helps himself to what he needs from your body, and this can sometimes mean that the mother will have some deficiency.

A fit and healthy body, supplemented by a healthy diet, is usually easily able to replenish any nutrients it might lack. This takes between three and nine months, hence the saying: nine months of pregnancy and nine months to recover from pregnancy. A body that is under stress, on the other hand, finds it harder to replenish the nutrients on its own. If your birth was traumatic you are probably producing a lot of stress hormones. These stress hormones make your digestion less efficient, which in turn means you absorb fewer nutrients. According to the health authorities, if your diet is healthy and varied you don't need to take extra vitamins or supplements. In my practice I've noticed that women do feel an enormous improvement from a short course of vitamin B-complex, vitamin D3, omega-3 or a multivitamin made especially for mothers. No matter how many physical complaints you may have or how tired you might be, it's important to keep moving. A simple exercise like a vigorous walk for half an hour in fresh air does wonders for your body and your mind.

Chronic pain

Some 7% of women still have chronic pain two years after giving birth. After having a baby you might have pain in your pelvis, your tailbone, your vagina, your anus, or the area between your vagina and your anus. The scars from a C-section, episiotomy or tear can be painful or you may experience stomach and back pain since the birth. It is unfortunately also very common to have pain while making love, leading to a host of consequences for your sex life.

Regrettably, chronic pain following childbirth is not discussed enough in the medical world and symptoms are often played down by doctors: *"That will pass on its own, it just needs time."* Women don't find it easy to talk about the pain either. They believe that nothing can be done about it, that "it's psychological", or that they are the only ones still experiencing pain after having their baby. The effect of chronic pain on your life can be huge. Pain makes you tired, it negatively influences the quality of your sleep and your lust for life, as well as limiting the way you function every day. Chronic pain can make you feel anxious or depressed. Above all, pain following childbirth reminds you continually of the birth. Always discuss (chronic) pain with your caregiver.

Lack of sleep: Mummy is tired!

Obviously in the first weeks after the arrival of your baby you will not sleep as you did before. You wake up for night feeds, hear every little sound your baby makes, and you might have engorged breasts or nightly sweats due to the hormonal changes. This is all normal and goes with the job of being new parents. However, some women can cope much better with lack of sleep than others. You probably know yourself how many hours of sleep you need. Take what you can get, whenever you can get it. A couple of extra hours in the evening or half an hour during the day can make all the difference. See if you and your partner can alternate with "night duty". It doesn't really make sense for the both of you to get up at night to feed and change the baby. Shared pain is half the pain unless you are both up all night. Very soon you will be so tired you will end up fighting like cats and dogs.

If you are breastfeeding it may seem like you are sleeping badly because your baby wants to drink a few times in the night. You are awake more often, but the good thing about breastfeeding is that you skip the first superficial stages of sleep and reach the deeper, more restorative stages more quickly. Because of this, you can get through the day with fewer hours of sleep. A hormonal cocktail of oxytocin (cuddling hormones), prolactin (caring hormones) and cholecystokinin (CCK, the sleeping hormone) helps you to feed your child while you are half asleep and then to fall asleep again easily. If you feel that you really aren't getting enough sleep and that the lack of sleep is stopping you from functioning during the day, you could consider sleeping in a separate room with ear plugs for a night. Sometimes one good night is enough to break the vicious circle of exhaustion. For that one night your partner can take over the feeds using expressed breastmilk. Of course, if you are using formula you can also let your partner take over the feeds while you have a night alone with your ear plugs.

Talk to your doctor if you keep suffering from nightmares about your birth experience or in which bad things happen to your baby. Nightmares may be a sign of PTSD. To find out if that's the case, you can start by writing down a description of your nightmare as it is, and then making up another – positive – ending. During the day, read the positive story. This will help you rewrite your nightmare. This method is called "rescripting". If this doesn't help you get rid of your nightmares it could be that something else is wrong. Talk to your doctor about the nightmares.

Concentration and memory problems

When women complain of being unable to concentrate, midwifes often reply, infuriatingly: *"Oh, that's just 'pregnancy brain'. It'll go away before the baby turns one."* But concentration problems can be a symptom of (postpartum) depression.
In that case, there is more to it than simply "pregnancy brain" or forgetfulness. You may not, for example, be able to read a book or to follow the plot of a film. You have difficulty listening to the person talking to you and you forget any appointments that you

have not written down. At work you are not as efficient as you used to be and you feel as though you are always playing catch-up. Your colleagues also notice that your concentration is low and your work suffers. If you have doubts about your ability to concentrate, ask your colleagues and your partner if they have noticed a difference and discuss it with your doctor.

An emotional rollercoaster or no emotions at all

The hormonal see-saw might make you react more emotionally after you give birth than you are used to. Some 70% of women have postpartum weeping in the first two weeks after giving birth. A distressing birth experience might leave you feeling like you are riding an emotional rollercoaster. You have a much shorter fuse than usual and can react in a hugely passionate way to the smallest, most insignificant thing. It seems like you can't bear anything. Anger, fury, frustration, irritation and sadness can lie just under the surface. It's normal to be prone to strong emotional reactions in the first six weeks after giving birth. If this lasts longer than six weeks, however, or if you don't recognize yourself or comprehend your reactions, speak to your doctor.

There are also women who don't feel any emotion at all as a result of a traumatic birth. Instead, they have a sort of emptiness, a lack of feeling. This can be a symptom of depression but also of PTSD. Your body might be so shaken from your birth experience that it goes into a sort of shut-down, a freeze mode, making you go around like an emotionless zombie. If you try to push away frightening images, thoughts or feelings, you might also be pushing away other feelings, to level things out. It's as if there is a heavy fire door blocking out your feelings. You can't easily access them. Picture it as a defence mechanism on the part of your brain. In doing this your brain ensures that you are not overwhelmed by frightening memories, thoughts and feelings.

"I work in the field of psychiatry and as a student was repeatedly told to keep my emotions under wraps and even to turn them off while I was at work. My birth experience was hellish and I recognised – through my work with traumatised patients – PTSD symptoms in myself. The GP and the work doctor confirmed my fears. I found it hard to accept that I was so emotional. For the smallest things tears would run down my cheeks, even while I was in conversation with patients. I also became unbelievably angry over the smallest things, my eyes would mist over. Working in those circumstances became impossible; I only managed six weeks following my maternity leave before I called in sick. What a failure: to work in the field of psychiatry and then to fall mentally ill myself! During the coaching sessions I processed not only my traumatic birth experience, I also learned that I was allowed to leave my emotions 'switched on' while I was at work. This was an eye opener. Of course, they are not as intense as during my PTSD episode, but I don't need to hide my emotions away anymore. If I'm moved during a discussion with a patient, I name the feeling and I might have a tear in my eye. I'm proud of this now because my patients go through a lot. In the end I came out of it stronger, even though I would much rather not have had a traumatic birth or PTSD. By daring to be vulnerable and to show my feelings it has become easier for my patients also to show their feelings. This improves the therapeutic relationship." (Veronica, 37 years old)

Brooding / ruminating

Many clients in my practice have – or shall we just say, suffer from – brooding thoughts and ruminations. The difference between thinking about something and brooding over it, is that when you think about something you align your thoughts until a solution appears and you can take action, whereas with brooding, your thoughts go around in circles: "What if...?", "If only I had...", "It could have...".

Thinking leads to action; brooding, on the other hand, paralyses you and leads to inaction. For this reason I liken brooding to cycling on a home trainer or on a swing, you spend a lot of energy on it but you don't move forward. Especially at night... everything looks worse and more hopeless at night. And you're so tired and you need your sleep so badly because in about two hours your baby is going to wake you for her next feed... it's normal to brood now and then, especially when there are big changes happening in your life, such as becoming a mother. It ceases to be normal when brooding takes over a large part of your day (and night!). In that case, brooding can be a symptom of anxiety or depression.

When you have had an unpleasant birth experience, there is a good chance you will worry over the way in which the birth went: "Why did the doctor...", "If only I had...", "Why didn't the midwife...", "Imagine if I had first..." It helps to write down your questions and to discuss them point by point with the midwife or gynaecologist who was present at the birth.

After speaking to the midwife or gynaecologist, if you still have periods of brooding, try the following exercise: for 30 days, brood over your experience as hard as you can twice a day for ten minutes. These two ten-minute periods are your brooding periods, once in the morning and once towards the end of the day. Choose the timing of your brooding periods yourself, but don't plan the second one after 9pm as it might stop you from falling asleep. Always finish the brooding period with a positive thought (focus on something that is going well) and with a short relaxation or breathing exercise (see page 75).

Make sure you are not disturbed during your brooding period and write down everything you are brooding over in a brooding diary. Outside of the brooding periods, jot down any new ruminations/brooding thoughts on a piece of paper. Fold up the paper and put it away. This act of folding and putting away symbolises your "parking the rumination". You leave the rumination "parked" until you're allowed to brood again in your designated ten-minute brooding period.

Say *"STOP, GO AWAY"* to brooding thoughts that come up in the meantime. In this way you train your brain that

YOU decide which thoughts are in YOUR head and on which thoughts you are going to spend your energy. Within a couple of weeks you will find that your brooding thoughts fade into the background. It becomes a lot easier for you to silence them.

If you are unable to "park" your brooding thoughts, or if you don't see an improvement even though you have been faithfully writing down your broods in your brooding diary, speak to your doctor. Explain what you have been doing and that you are still suffering from the brooding. The doctor can refer you to a psychologist or coach specialised in cognitive behavioural therapy (see Chapter 8).

Compensating for your insecurity with the urge to be in control

The arrival of a child is overwhelming and brings a period of insecurity for most parents. All those involved (including the baby) need to find a new balance. It's normal to feel the need to be in control more during this period, especially because you feel you have no control over the situation. Often, the more insecure you are and the less (self-)confidence you have, the greater your need to control things becomes. But you can't always do everything perfectly. There's no such thing as a perfect mother!

Perfectionism often stems from insecurity. Insecurity is often the result of a fear of rejection. Everyone has this fear to some extent. We all need to feel that we belong and that we're accepted. The fear of rejection is stoked by the fear that we aren't good enough as we are. The more insecure you are, the less you trust yourself. Insecurity and a lack of (self-)confidence can be caused by (or can lead to) a negative self-image.
A negative birth experience and the feeling during the birth that you lost all control can throw you into an urge to be controlling. That urge can quickly become a compulsion to be controlling.

An exercise to improve your self-image
Ask different people around you, such as your partner, a friend, colleague, sister, mother (-in-law) or (former) study mate, how they see you. Each one will know a different side of you because each one has a different connection with you in a different context. Some of my clients perk up enormously when they find out how positively they are viewed by the people around them. Complete the following self-image exercise. It will hopefully help you to improve your self-image and to reduce your need to be in control.

1. Which negative words do you use when you think about yourself? A negative self-image often involves the following themes: looks, social success, intelligence, social skills.

2. Name a few situations/examples where you "messed up". In other words, what is the concrete evidence that validates the negative statements you made about yourself above?

3. How did you come up with these negative conclusions about yourself? Who gave you this label, and at what point in your life? What do you do, or allow, as a result of the negative statements you made about yourself above?

4. What do you feel and in which part of your body do you feel it, when you think negatively about yourself or when you answer the questions above? (For example, shivers, tension, heaviness.)

5. How would you like to think about yourself? Try to translate the points you answered to question 1 into their opposites, or at least a neutral counterpart. If you answered "I'm not good enough" to question 1, you can now say "I'm okay" or "I am good enough".

6. Which body language, facial expression and voice fit your desired self-image?

7. Who do you know who could serve as a role model for you? Who do you know who exhibits that behaviour?
Try to imagine how your role model would react to different situations. What would he/she say in those cases? What can you learn from that? What could you do differently?

8. Can you name some examples or situations in which you

did or were what you wanted to do or be? When were you "good", "fun", "attractive", "smart" or "nice" enough? Who were you with? Where were you? How did you feel? What did you do?

9. Which – short, powerful and positive – statement can you choose as a mantra? Which positive image of yourself (see question 5) goes with it? What kind of body language, facial expression and voice (see question 6) go with it?

"Since Bas was born I've been out of balance. I don't actually really understand why I feel unhappy. I have an extremely kind husband, an exemplary baby, a beautiful house, a pleasant family and family-in-law, many friends and a great job with great colleagues. Unfortunately, my head is stuffed much too full with everything that I would like to organise perfectly. I want to bring up my son perfectly, he mustn't miss out on anything and everything must go according to the textbook. I would like to give my husband enough attention, as I'm afraid he'll leave me if I don't. I want to keep my house perfectly clean and tidy so that we can have a pleasant and healthy life in it. The amount of work I do has remained the same, except that now I'm cramming five days' worth of work into four days. In addition I have my social life and regular exercise on my wish list (or rather, 'must-do list'), because I'm worried I won't lose my pregnancy weight otherwise.

Bas's arrival made me lose control of my life. He was born three weeks early and I was not emotionally ready for him. In my head I knew he could come from 37 weeks onwards but it felt too early for me. Because I felt that I had lost control, I turned into a control freak. I saw myself doing it but I couldn't help it. I even gave instructions to the crèche, as if they didn't know how to look after a baby. At work I drove my colleagues mad with my need to control everything. Until then I had had blind faith in them, and suddenly now I found myself checking all the outgoing post. This made me get late with my other tasks, so that I had to work even harder to keep my grip. I was heading straight for a burnout. During the coaching sessions I understood that I felt like a failure if things (pretty much everything) didn't happen the way I had planned in my head. Everyone said I shouldn't put the bar so high but the message didn't come through. I could only see what didn't go right. When I finally saw for myself how compulsively I was behaving – I'm not like that! – I was able to change. My mantra became 'good is good enough' and slowly I started to get better." (Amira, 28 years old)

Fear / anxiety

It's completely normal to feel some anxiety in a new (life) situation. Fear makes us alert and ensures that we can react quickly in emergencies. Some 12% of pregnant women and new mothers feel anxious in the year they become mothers. More than half of these women experience these complaints for the first time in their lives. A good 80% of these anxiety symptoms go unnoticed by doctors because women don't easily speak of their thoughts and feelings of anxiety. If you don't talk about it, the symptoms can worsen. It helps to face your feelings of anxiety and dare to share them. Being a little anxious and extra careful is fine, but to let your life be influenced by fear is not. I like to distinguish between fear of real obstacles (rational *fear*) and imaginary ones (irrational *anxiety*). The first type of fear leads to action, the second type paralyses. When you're afraid, your body gets ready to fight or escape *(flight)*. Your heart rate increases, you breathe more quickly, your blood pressure rises, your digestion slows down and your muscles get ready for extra exertion. But what happens if that exertion doesn't need to be used? You remain super-alert and tense because of the catastrophes that potentially might happen.

Your heart rate and breathing remain high and your body exhausts itself from the over-alert fight-or-flight mode. It produces excessive stress hormones in order to stay alert and in the long term this exhausts you. You can also become extra anxious because of your high heart rate and quick breathing, forcing you into a vicious circle which leaves you at risk of panic attacks. How can you differentiate between anxious and over-anxious? If you regularly have a bad premonition, as if something bad is about to happen, or if you are nervous and worried without there being a reason/cause you can point at, you are probably more anxious than is good for you.

If you're unable to relax and your body often feels tense (in your neck, shoulders, back and stomach), and you notice that you avoid people and situations because you're afraid bad things will happen, there should be alarm bells. Talk to your doctor about your fears.

Depression

Between 10% and 25% of new parents (mothers and fathers!) suffer from feelings of depression in the first year following the birth of their child. This new phase of life is so different that parents may need between a couple of months and a year to adjust to the new situation. It's normal to feel glum and down now and then, to sleep badly, to lose your appetite occasionally or to lack energy. However, if you have these symptoms several weeks in a row and they negatively affect your life on a daily basis or several days per week, you may be suffering from depression.

Research shows that more than 50% of women with established PTSD have depression. Women who suffer from depression during pregnancy have a higher chance of experiencing a traumatic birth and developing PTSD symptoms. Here again, speak to your GP about your complaints.

Burnout

If you continuously hold a rubber band taut it will eventually snap. It's normal to feel stressed for a while when you're in a new phase in your life. However, if you find it hard to relax and have physical complaints such as headaches, backache, stomach aches or heart palpitations, you are in the danger zone. You go from being tense to being drained and if you then keep ignoring the signals from your body, you can become overstrained or have a burnout.

New parents are, in any case, more susceptible to burnout. The pressure is high and there is hardly a moment to recharge either at work or at home. If you just keep on going without listening to your body, there will come a moment when your body calls for a halt. The number one symptom of a burnout is a feeling of total exhaustion. Other symptoms are difficulty concentrating and remembering things, anxiety and panic attacks, sleeping problems, a feeling of haste and being over-alert, or feeling down and depressed.

If you have PTSD complaints you are almost twice as likely to have a burnout. Imagine how exhausting it would be to be alert to possible danger 24/7. Nobody is able to keep that up. If you think you or your partner might be at risk of a burnout, ask your GP or company doctor for help.

Often, the earlier you spot the problem, the faster you will recover. Try to get your rest, when and where you can. Yoga, meditation and mindfulness can help you relax and to live in the NOW, instead of thinking and planning ten steps ahead. The tips at the end of this chapter can also help you to curb a looming burnout or to recover from a burnout.

Negative sexual experiences

Regrettably, the figures relating to negative sexual experiences are shocking. Almost half of women have a negative sexual experience before the age of 20. The abuser is often a family member. Although it's well known that negative sexual experiences have a big impact, there has hardly been any research on the impact of a distressing birth experience on a person who has previously suffered abuse. This is because women find it hard to talk about being sexually abused in the past or about their negative sexual experiences. Many midwives ask specifically about this, but many women are unwilling or unable to answer honestly. They are happy to be pregnant and don't want to be confronted again with negative sexual experiences from their past. Suppressed memories of sexual experiences can resurface due to traumatic childbirth, because your physical and psychological boundaries are crossed once again. If this happens to you, if giving birth brings back painful memories of sexual abuse, ask for extra coaching.

"I hated it but acted as if I was enjoying it. Everyone fell for my pretence; everyone, except my newborn son. He smiled for his father and for his sister, but never for me. When I was changing him he turned his head away from me. I became increasingly listless, I felt empty inside and soon people started noticing. I wasn't able to concentrate at work and made one mistake after another. I ended up home with postnatal depression. When I spoke to my coach about the birth and the helplessness I had felt, I began to gag. I explained that I felt disgusted with myself because I hadn't stood up for myself and that I found it disgusting that the doctor continued with the ventouse while I was screaming 'STOP!'

The coach observed that I spoke of 'disgust' a few times in my story. She asked if the birth might have brought back memories of other 'disgusting' things. The question gave me flashbacks to my youth, where disgusting things had indeed taken place. Things that I had buried so deeply that I had (almost) forgotten them. Things I had never mentioned to anyone. The memories flooded back with a vengeance. After a couple of sessions she referred me to a therapist specialising in sexual abuse, with whom I followed very intensive treatment for a year and a half. It was a very intense period and there were times when I wished that I had been able to keep burying the memories, but I could also see that that was stopping me from living fully. With hindsight, I can see that the traumatic birth enabled me to face and process past traumas. I also received extra coaching for my relationship with my baby and we are now functioning much better as a family." (Marion, 41 years old)

Postpartum psychosis (PPP)

Postpartum psychosis is a psychosis that comes about in the first month(s) after giving birth. The chance of PPP is luckily very small: 1 to 2 in 1,000. A woman with PPP can be a danger to herself and to her baby, so professional help is necessary and there is often (forced) hospitalisation in specialised care. The mother is increasingly restless, suspicious, irritable and confused. This often goes hand in hand with – and is made worse by – lack of sleep. She might have delusions and hallucinations. Science has not yet found a link between traumatic childbirth and PPP.

What you can do yourself to aid your psychological and physical recovery

In this chapter you have read what the consequences can be of an (unprocessed) distressing birth experience on yourself, your health and your work/career. Unfortunately, the consequences aren't limited to you, they can also negatively impact your relationship with your baby and with your partner. You can read more about that in Chapters 4 and 5.

To conclude this chapter, here are some tips and exercises:

1. **Every day, do some medium intensity exercise for at least 30 minutes.**
   Vegetating on the couch because you're too tired to exercise has the opposite effect of what you want. (Outdoor) exercise causes your brain to produce happy chemicals (endorphins). Medium intensity exercise means walking fast rather than jogging. You can join specially designed outdoor programmes such as a boot camp for mums, or you can just walk strenuously while pushing the pram, no matter the weather. If you ask a friend to join you, you kill two birds with one stone. An apt Buddhist saying goes: Take half an

hour every day for relaxation/meditation or a nature walk. Unless you are busy, in that case take one hour.

2. **Social contact**
   Make sure you have enough social contact. People who are depressed have a tendency to withdraw and to avoid social contact because they – incorrectly – assume that friends are not waiting for them because they don't have anything fun to say. By going for a walk with a friend, you break through the unsociable behaviour that is characteristic of depression. Spending time with happy people makes you happy too. A happy person in your immediate surroundings increases your own feeling of happiness by 10%!

3. **Relaxation exercises and massage**
   In the morning before you get up and in the evening as you're going to bed, do a relaxation exercise. This is extra important because your body and your muscles are tense if you've undergone a distressing event. The tenser you are, the shorter your fuse will be. A relaxation exercise will help you begin the day in a more relaxed way, so that you don't lose your cool so easily, and to end the day feeling more relaxed, letting you sleep better. A massage can work wonders to help relax tensed muscles. Ask your partner or a friend to massage you or go to a specialised (pregnancy) masseuse.

4. **Breathing exercises**
   The National Centre for Stress Management has developed the breathing guidance app *Respiroguide Pro*, which is based on the most recent research into neuroscience and stress management. The app helps you to optimise the frequency of your breathing rhythm. You help your body to relax by regulating your breathing. This brings your autonomous nervous system to a restful state and changes your heart rhythm. Your basic heart rate slows and the variability of your heart rhythm increases. This is known as

cardiac coherence. This interplay between your breathing and your heart can be compared to being on a swing. By giving yourself a little push (with your breathing) you get into a pleasant swinging rhythm. With your breathing you give your heart the correct push. For my patients (and for myself) I use a slightly more extensive device (emWave Pro from Heartmath), which uses biofeedback via a sensor on your earlobe to plot your heart rate and cardiac coherence on a computer chart.

5. **Mindfulness and meditation**
   Mindfulness (attention training), yoga and meditation can help you monitor your thoughts with gentleness and compassion. Your thoughts come and go. You are not your thoughts; they just drop by for a visit in your brain. How much attention you give them is up to you. The more attention you give them the more "real" they become, the more weight there is attached to them. Mindfulness can help you to turn inwards and to observe, without judgment, the thoughts and sensations in your body. It's a question of practise, practise, practise. Nowadays we have so much stimulation to deal with compared with two generations ago (the generation of our grandparents). Even when we're on holiday the stream of messages and stimuli continues.
   If you are under stress because of a difficult labour, it's much harder to cope with all the stimuli and you become even more stressed. (Social media) silence can then be a blessing for your busy mind.
   You can join a (group) course or use videos or apps at home to practise mindfulness, yoga or meditation.

6. **Water the roses, not the thistles**
   There's a saying: "If you give attention to something, it will grow". If you focus on all the things that are not going well in your life, you only strengthen your negative feelings and there is a good chance you will become more depressed. Give attention to the things that make you grow and hopefully

blossom again. Concretely, you can approach this in three ways (or four, if you have an iPhone). Choose the way that appeals most to you, or use a combination of all of them.

a) Make a list of things you enjoyed before your pregnancy, and do one of them every day. Stick with small things such as buying a magazine, drinking coffee on an outdoor terrace, soaking in the bath for a while, treating yourself to a bunch of flowers, enjoying some time alone, a shopping trip, going out for dinner or a film with your partner or a friend or starting to exercise again.

b) Keep a diary of "nice things" or "things-I'm-thankful-for". Every day, jot down things that you were happy about, that went well, that you're proud of or thankful for. Try to list at least three things every day. Even if you didn't have a good day at all, try to think of three highlights. Within a couple of weeks, this should make you feel more positive.

c) Take a photo every day of a fun moment or something you're grateful for. You probably have a mobile phone on you most of the time. When you see something special, no matter how insignificant, immortalise it. Store the photos in a special folder or post them to Instagram or Pinterest. When you're feeling down, you can look back at these photos of cheerful moments.

d) If you have an iPhone you can buy the *MoodMint* app (it's not yet available for other phones, unfortunately). The app consists of a scientifically designed game that lasts one minute each time. You can play it as often as you like, for a minimum of five times a day. In that minute you need to choose the most positive of four pictures as fast as you can. In this way you train your brain to focus on the positive (the roses). This is very useful for people with depression who tend to focus on negative things (the thistles) and on what is wrong with their lives.

Karishma's

I was so happy to be pregnant, at least until I reached 32 weeks. I felt great, everyone said I looked radiant, my husband thought I was beautiful and at work everything was going well. In the last weeks of my pregnancy I suddenly developed high blood pressure. When I was 38 and a half weeks pregnant the gynaecologist decided to induce labour the following day. I was disappointed but thought, if it's necessary, then we should do it. I had been very relaxed throughout my pregnancy, I had prepared myself for the birth by doing yoga and I was looking forward to getting the birth over with! On the first day of the induction procedure, my husband and I had laughed a lot and the time flew by. In the evening my husband went to visit his parents because his father had just had an operation. Suddenly, at 1am, I was woken up by pain in my stomach. I started timing the pains on my mobile phone and called the nurse. She told me I wasn't having real contractions yet, and there was no need to call my husband. She advised me to sleep some more as I would need my energy the next day for the delivery. I was already collapsing from the pain and she wanted me to sleep? I felt like a small child who had been reprimanded.

In the hours after that, I found myself crawling on the floor from the pain. If this was "nothing", how on earth was I to cope tomorrow when the "real contractions" started? I felt terribly alone, on the floor in the labour room. I needed to be sick but the cramps made it too painful for me to stand up and go to the bathroom. I was sick on the floor and cleaned it up as best I could between contractions using paper towels. What a nightmare! I didn't dare call the nurse again, I didn't want to be a drama queen. The nurse came in only after a couple of hours. She found me on the floor on my hands and knees and apparently also saw how desperate I was because she asked: *"Why didn't you call?"* For the second time I felt like I had been scolded, I had got it wrong again. I had failed twice, before the real exam had even properly begun.

The nurse went to consult with the doctor. I was only one centimetre dilated and he thought it was too soon for an epidural. Instead I was given an injection of painkillers and sleeping medication. This threw me completely out of it. Every time I had a contraction I felt like I needed to wrestle my way above water while the sheets on my legs pulled me back down again. Then I was hit by a particularly intense contraction and I slipped away again into unconsciousness. A couple of hours later I was three centimetres dilated and they called my husband. I was happy that I wouldn't be alone anymore, but because of the medication I wasn't really present and my husband couldn't do very much for me anyway. According to the doctor, the shot was to help me relax but it only made me anxious.

In the morning I couldn't take it anymore and I asked for an epidural again, only to be told by the gynaecologist that my labour had progressed too far for an epidural. He thought it wouldn't be long before I would need to start pushing. That gave me hope. But it took hours more before I was completely dilated. I felt like I had been tricked. By the end of the morning the doctor said there was just a rim left and that he would hold that back so I could push the head out past it. It wasn't quite clear to me what was happening. It was different from what I had learned in my pregnancy yoga class. I hadn't had the really strong contractions they had talked about. The doctor's hand, holding back the last edge was more painful. I felt like I was just doing anything. They kept saying *"good, you're doing well"*, but after an hour, it wasn't so convincing. They asked if perhaps I wasn't daring to push. This made me feel for the third time like I had failed the birthing exam. After an hour and a half of pushing, I was completely exhausted. The baby was still too high up for the ventouse but they still wanted to try. There was a growing chance I would need a caesarean. I didn't care anymore, I only thought: get that child out of me NOW and leave me in peace.

The ventouse appeared and was violently pushed inside me. I saw my partner looking away. I heard a strange noise – I couldn't make sense of everything I was hearing. My eyes were closed but I could hear everything. I pushed with all my might while the doctor pulled with all his might. Nothing happened. I felt the doctors begin to panic because they couldn't get any further. Suddenly the nurse pressed very hard on my stomach. The gynaecologist said I *"had to give it everything I had"* and shouted *"push, push!"* At the same time he pulled on the pump/ventouse. I was thinking, they are either going to break my baby or me! It was dreadful! At last she was born, with an unbelievable pointy head. I thought: I really hope that gets better. Sheela cried immediately. My husband told me later that the umbilical cord had been wrapped around her neck a couple of times and they first had to cut through it. The ordeal was over and Sheela didn't seem to have suffered. She lay watching me with wide-open eyes. I looked back at her, dazed by the brutality I had just been through. They still had to stitch me up and I gave our daughter to my husband to hold. I was afraid of dropping her and thus failing for the fourth time during my labour. The stitches took forever, I just let it all come over me as if I wasn't really there. In the meantime, Sheela had fallen asleep in her father's arms. It looked so natural, my husband as a father with his daughter in his arms. He could clearly do it, I obviously could not.

The first days went well enough. The nurse was kind and patient. She tried to calm me down. I heard what she said but secretly still compared it to when I was in labour. Then, they had also told me I was doing well, but eventually they had needed a pump and lots of pushing and pulling for my baby to be able to be born. The fourth day was "daddy-day". My husband bathed our daughter and was complimented by the nurse and by the visitors who came by that day. He was the perfect father, even I could see that. I, on the other hand, felt lost. I trembled on my feet and the breastfeeding was clearly not going well either because our daughter had lost almost 10% of her weight. My husband had to give her extra bottles of milk. She gulped them down – the poor child was hungry.

A few weeks later I had recovered physically but I was still far from being my old self. Every noise made me jump, every unexpected movement, anything that didn't go as planned. I constantly hovered over my daughter and was over-protective. I was terribly unsure of myself, I dithered constantly and had turned into a scared little mouse. I preferred to stay safely indoors as much as possible. I put friends and colleagues off from visiting with excuses and saw almost nobody. It felt as though my husband and I lived in two separate worlds. His world was more or less the same as before he became a father; he went to work and fitted fatherhood very naturally into his free time. My own life had changed beyond recognition since giving birth. I stayed locked up at home, half panicking, and unable to look after my baby or myself. I brooded day and night over everything I had done wrong. I was afraid my husband would leave me. He kept asking when I was going to be myself again, how long this was going to last, and regretted that he didn't know anymore how he could cheer me up. Everything he said irritated me because he often said precisely what I didn't want to hear – especially not from him.

I felt like I had failed during the birth and now I was failing at being a mother. I was jealous when my friends talked about their birth experiences. I envied how radiant they were just after giving birth and how naturally they seemed to be able to look after their babies. In one of my first coaching sessions I did an exercise to change my feeling from one of failure to one of mere annoyance about what had happened to me. This made a world of difference to me. For four months I had blamed myself for everything. I felt I had failed at giving birth and at being a mother, as well as as a wife and employee. After doing the exercise, I felt annoyed about the way in which the birth went, but I also felt that it wasn't just my fault. What a relief! I felt my shoulders loosen up and I noticed I was breathing more deeply and calmly. The coach also advised my husband to write down his own experience of the birth, after which we read each other's versions. They were really two very different accounts of the same birth. No wonder we couldn't understand each other. We also went to the coach together a couple of times. She acted as an "interpreter" between us so that we could understand how we had lost each other following the birth. Together with her we could talk to each other without it escalating. In one session we literally had to change places and tell the story as the other had experienced it. This gave us more understanding for each other. We also learned how we – often accidently but sometimes purposely – pressed each other's "red button" and how we could ask for a time-out if one of us got too close to the other's red button.

During the sessions I realised that the worst memory was the part where I was alone on all fours, throwing up on the floor and when the nurse came in and told me that this was "nothing". I could still remember that feeling of being completely alone. The feeling that I was not being taken seriously was also very painful. I realised that I had maintained part of the loneliness after the birth when I clammed up and didn't let anyone in on my thoughts. Because of this I kept feeling lonely and was gradually slipping away. The part where I got the morphine shot and the helpless state it left me in was another low point. By writing down my ruminations twice a day for ten minutes in a notebook meant that within three weeks I spent much less time ruminating and had more energy. My husband and I started to do fun things together as before and I went out with my friends again. Slowly I started to get my life back.

In one of the last sessions I "re-enacted" the birth, this time as I would have liked it to happen: with my husband by my side the whole time, without the morphine that made me feel so awful. I stood up for myself. This turned out to be the turning point. I realised that I had been dependent on others my whole life. My mother is the sweetest mother I could hope for, but she always did everything for me. This made me very dependent on her. I was still very much my mother's child – how could I be a mother to a child of my own? I have now created some distance from my mother and become closer to my partner. Sheela's arrival has changed several aspects of my life. Without the horrible birth experience I might never have realised that. Nowadays I am happy again at work, my husband and I get on well again and we're happy to be with each other and with our baby daughter.

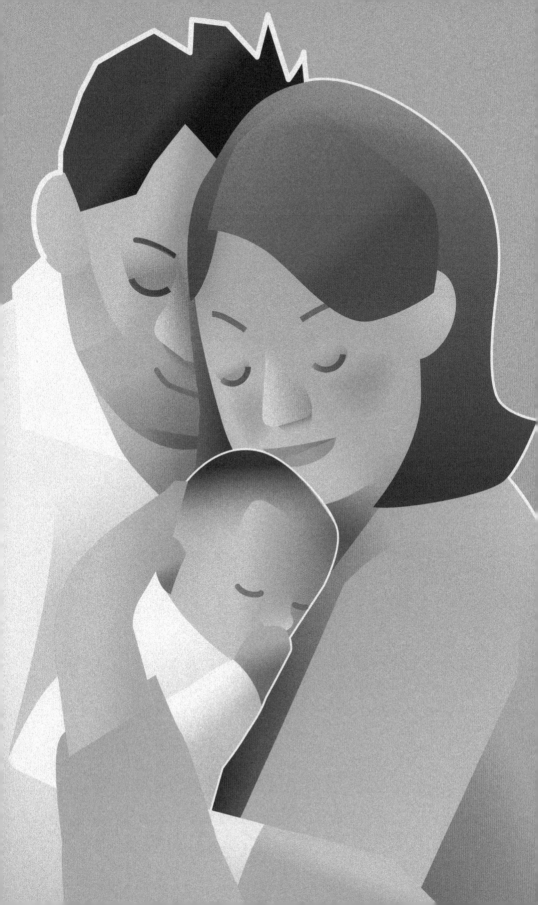

CHAPTER 4

A distressing birth
– how it affects your baby

As you can probably imagine, if you've had a bad birth experience and still feel the effects of it, your baby will also be affected. Before you begin to read this chapter, I'd like to warn you: it can be painful to read. Not only have you just been through a distressing birth, you feel "out of balance" and now you are reading about what the effects are on your baby. I'm not writing this to give you something to feel concerned or guilty about. You can't do anything about the fact that your birth experience was distressing. It happened to you, it isn't your fault. What you can do – and this is why I have included this chapter in the book – is to take action to limit the consequences of the distressing birth on your child and your family.

The importance of a strong bond

During pregnancy, your baby develops faster than at any other time in his life. In the space of nine months, two miniscule cells grow to become a complete tiny person. A baby cannot take care of himself and is therefore completely dependent on the care of his parents or guardians, with whom he instinctively tries to form an attachment from the moment of birth. This process of forming an emotional attachment is called bonding. The stronger the bond, the greater the chance of an optimal start in life for your child. If you as a parent are having trouble keeping yourself together emotionally or if you don't feel well psychologically, it's understandable that you won't be completely available to respond to your baby. You are, understandably, preoccupied with yourself. But if you aren't emotionally available, reachable or involved enough for your child, whom can your baby turn to?

In 2014, the *1001 Critical Days manifesto* was set up in the United Kingdom and became a political agenda point. This manifesto puts forward that the first 1001 days in a human life, from conception until the child is two years old, is the most crucial period of development in a child's life. In this period, a million (!) new connections are made per second (!) in the brain. The better and more safely a child can bond with his parents in this period, the greater the chance of the "best possible life". The more guidance the child and – where needed or desired – his parents get in that period, the smaller the chance of severe psychological, socio-emotional, developmental or learning problems the child will have later in life. The manifesto advocates prevention and early intervention. This means that parents and young children receive guidance where necessary at a very early stage. Currently, children are usually referred to a specialist once they have problems at school. If these problems stem from parent-child bonding issues, the negative interaction patterns are already engraved and the child is already unsafely bonded, with all the consequences thereof.

"I knew I hadn't been well emotionally since I gave birth to my third child. Our third child needs special care because he has a birth defect. The labour went very quickly, but the baby's heartbeat dropped away completely at the end and the doctors began to panic, making it a frightening experience. As soon as he was born, Tim was taken by the paediatrician and was kept in the children's ward. Tim's birth defect has nothing to do with the delivery but I had unconsciously still connected the two things in my head. I resented him for upsetting the balance in our family, and for all the extra care he needed; that since his arrival I was unable to keep all the balls in the air. Until he came into it, our life was perfectly ordered, in every respect. Why had I wanted a third child so badly?

Forcing myself to look back at Tim's birth and the feelings I had then was both painful and liberating. I thought I was a terrible mother because I was so angry at Tim, because I resented him for sowing confusion into our lives. I learned that my anger was normal. At one point, I took a dinner service – especially bought for this purpose –

and smashed it to pieces while crying uncontrollably about the whole situation. After that, I felt less angry, less tense. The birth was something I had undergone, it wasn't pleasant but I no longer had nightmares about it. Tim belonged in our family. His disability is not nice, but he is nice. I learned to see Tim separately from his disability and this enabled me to see other sides to him.

I learned to massage Tim and this gave us a much more positive way of being together. I saw him relax while I massaged him and it made me relax too. The more relaxed he was, the more he smiled and the less he cried. The sound of his crying also changed: it was much less piercing. My coach said this was because I was changing too. My nerves, which had been at their most sensitive since the birth, began to relax and this made it easier for me to accept his crying. I also got a massage once a week in that period and I faithfully did my relaxation exercises twice a day. Slowly I clambered out of the rut I'd been stuck in and my family clambered out with me.

My partner and I had some couple therapy sessions too. This enabled us to have more understanding for each other. We were dealing with Tim's disability in different ways. My husband had a much more practical approach: while I wanted to talk about it, he came up with solutions and advice. During the therapy sessions we learned to listen to each other better and to understand why each of us reacted in the way we did. Since then, we've learned to take a time-out before an argument escalates. We noticed that our eldest daughter, who is a very sensitive child, started bringing friends over to play at our house again. For the first two years after Tim was born she hadn't wanted to, probably because the atmosphere was so tense at home.

I resigned from my job and now do freelance work from home. This works much better to accommodate our family life and the extra care that Tim needs." (Madeleine, 35 years old)

It takes a village to raise a child

Families are much smaller than they used to be. Because of this, children have much fewer siblings from whom they can learn and for whom they can serve as an example or role model. Families are also much more inwardly focused than before. In a sense, they have retreated behind their own front door. Children play outdoors much less and extended families spend less time together because everyone is busy.

They say it takes a village to raise a child. Nowadays, however, most families seem to be living on an (otherwise deserted) island rather than in a close village community where the parental tasks are shared. It also means that when things aren't going smoothly on the "island" the child doesn't have alternative models. When both parents aren't comfortable emotionally, they mirror each other and the stress level in the home rises tangibly. Two parents with short fuses are quicker to argue and to become irritated with their children's behaviour. Even if the arguments play out in the evenings when the children are in bed, the children can sense much more tension in a family than the adults realise. Growing up in a house full of tension and hostility is disastrous for a child and undermines a safe bonding process as well as the building of a strong self-image.

"We hadn't been together very long when I had an unplanned pregnancy. My boyfriend wanted me to terminate it but I didn't want that. My refusal surprised me because I hadn't necessarily wanted to have a child before. Since I refused to have an abortion, my boyfriend decided to end our relationship. The pregnancy went well, but the delivery was terrible. I felt that I was not at all taken seriously as a young, single mother. They treated me as if I was less capable than others. Because of that I felt a stronger urge to prove myself as a mother.

My whole life revolved around Noa. I hardly saw my friends anymore. I only left Noa with my mother when I had to go to work, and then I gave my mother a detailed list of what Noa needed and at exactly what time. Every day, there was something that hadn't gone exactly as I had specified on my list and then I had a row with my mother. I felt such a sense of responsibility for Noa. I wanted to be her mother and her father as well as her best friend. I didn't let her miss out on anything, everything had to be perfectly organised.

I learned to ask for help. My coach called it *'granting your friends a helper's high'*. My friends told me they had really felt like I had shut them out. I never gave them a chance to form a bond with Noa. I thought they were completely uninterested in my life as a mother, when in fact it turned out many of my friends loved to babysit. This allowed me to get some exercise or to have an evening out. Things were going much better for me until about a week before Noa's first birthday. I couldn't understand what was happening because I had been looking forward to her birthday. By coincidence I had a coaching session that week. The coach explained that our bodies have a memory for unpleasant events and this was going to be the anniversary of my unpleasant birth experience. Apparently this is called the 'anniversary effect.' It was my body telling me it was time to process the birth. I did this using a special exercise: pretending I could erase the bad delivery and replace it with a more positive story. And it worked too. I realised my fear of not being taken seriously was a recurring theme in my life. As a result of this realisation, my need to prove myself as a woman and as a mother also became less compulsive." (Demi, 23 years old)

Children do what you do, not what you say!

Through you, your child learns to understand herself, her environment, other people and the world. You facilitate, your child learns. Through you, as a parent, your child also learns how to deal with her emotions, impressions and tensions.

There are four basic emotions: happy, afraid, angry and sad
The better you're able to handle your emotions, the better you can teach your child to handle hers. Were you allowed to be angry, afraid or sad when you were a child?

| Happy | Afraid | Angry | Sad |

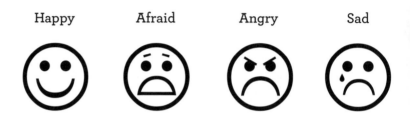

"My parents are wonderful, but when I was growing up it was considered unsociable to be angry and if I was sad, I was told to pull myself together. They had been taught this in turn by their own parents. I was faced with all sorts of negative emotions and frustrations since giving birth and becoming a mother. The more irritated I got, the more annoying my son became (and vice versa). I was often infuriated with him, and then I heard that at nursery he played sweetly with the other children and listened obediently to the teachers. It seemed like he was a different child there than when he was home. I became more and more insecure. The turning point came when I began to feel my emotions and also let them show. That helped me and my son. He used to have violent tantrums, but since he learned to take his frustration out by punching a cushion, he hasn't had them anymore. Punching cushions also helped me to ease my frustration. I sometimes also screamed and cried in the shower, with the music on full volume so that nobody could hear me. This provided some relief. One time, when I was getting angry with him, my son brought me a cushion himself. We each took turns to pummel the cushion until we were both in fits of giggles. It was a fantastic moment." (Cath, 33 years old)

If your child learns from you that he's okay, that you, his parent, are okay and can be trusted, that other people are okay and the world is okay to live in, he will develop a strong sense of confidence and resilience to go about discovering the world. When faced with a setback, he will likely react with: "It went wrong this time, I've learned from it, it will be better next time." He will feel "annoyance" (the fault of the circumstances) instead of "failure" (my fault, I've failed).

If you or your partner is rigid with tension (your system has been struck by lightning) or if one of you has been feeling down following a bad birth experience, you will behave differently from the way you normally do. Your reactions might be steered by anxiety, you might be more irritable and more prone to arguing than you were before the birth. You have enough to deal with with your own feelings. The feelings of your baby and those of your partner are too much to think about. You think you're failing as a parent. Your baby's crying or behaviour irritates you. You feel that your partner, parents or healthcare providers let you down during the birth, didn't take you seriously or even caused you pain or upset.

Because your baby senses whatever you're thinking or feeling, he will learn the following from you:

- **I'm not okay.** If I cry my mother/father gets angry at me or walks away from me instead of holding me, cuddling and comforting me or feeding or changing me. It must be my fault.
- **My mother/father is not okay.** She/he reacts angrily or dismissively when I cry. She/he doesn't understand what I'm trying to convey, doesn't respond when I smile, babble or try to make contact, so I'll stop doing it.
- **Other people are not okay.** My mother/father is apparently

afraid of them, keeps her/his distance from them and is sullen or aggressive when she/he interacts with them.

- **The world is not okay.** My parents keep telling me to "look out, be careful", so the world must be a very dangerous place. My parents don't look forward to new things or to meeting new people, so those must be unpleasant experiences. My parents feel upset when they hear about the news, the world economy and wars, so the world must be unpleasant and unsafe, maybe even terrible.

Communicating and making contact with your baby

Babies communicate fully with you, even without words. As parents, you discover together what every cry means. When does the baby want to eat? When and how does she want to be comforted? Which cry indicates that he's in pain? Your baby is trying to give you a message. And by learning from your mistakes you will figure out her instruction manual. Feeling helpless on the way is completely normal. It's extremely frustrating when you notice that what worked well with your elder child does nothing or even has the opposite effect with the younger one. Luckily, most parents find their way through the woods together. Unfortunately, it's much harder if you yourself are very tense, anxious, sad or depressed as a result of a distressing birth and the PTSD symptoms that sprang from it. You'll have less energy for your baby and you can't bring yourself to put yourself in his position; you can barely put yourself in your own position. There is a danger that you and your baby will end up in a vicious circle of not understanding each other and irritating each other.

If you don't understand your baby, he won't learn to understand himself and this will increase his frustration. A baby expresses frustration by crying, a toddler by throwing tantrums.

If you feel depressed or anxious following a traumatic birth experience, your facial expression will also be affected. You smile less and the corners of your mouth are more often turned downwards. When you smile, your eyes don't smile with your mouth. The baby picks up on this perfectly. Your choice of words is different, you use fewer words and the tone of your voice doesn't go up at the end of a sentence. You initiate less eye contact with the baby. When your baby smiles at you, you might miss the signal and not smile back. If your baby babbles, you don't babble back. If she claps her hands, you don't compliment her on it. You may not even hear it, because your thoughts are elsewhere, because you are brooding. But when a baby notices that her mother (or father) doesn't respond when she's trying to make contact, she will gradually give up trying to get your attention. She will shut herself off from her parents, to spare herself the pain and grief that comes with rejection.

The following questions are based on the Postpartum Bonding Questionnaire developed by Brockington.

1.	I feel close to my baby.	yes / no
2.	I love to cuddle my baby.	yes / no
3.	I can usually comfort my baby.	yes / no
4.	I enjoy playing/spending time with my baby.	yes / no
5.	I'm proud of my baby.	yes / no
6.	I love my baby.	yes / no
7.	I understand what my baby wants when he cries.	yes / no
8.	I feel confident when changing my baby.	yes / no
9.	I trust myself as a parent.	yes / no
10.	I see myself as this baby's parent. It feels "right".	yes / no
11.	I wish the old days, when I had no baby, would come back.	yes / no
12.	I regret having this baby.	yes / no

13. My baby winds me up/irritates me.	yes / no
14. I feel like this isn't my baby or that this baby doesn't belong with me.	yes / no
15. I feel trapped as a parent.	yes / no
16. I feel angry with my baby.	yes / no
17. I wish my baby would somehow go away.	yes / no
18. I'm afraid of my baby.	yes / no
19. I feel like hurting my baby/silencing my baby.	yes / no
20. I think my baby cries just to annoy me/ bothers me on purpose.	yes / no

If you answered 'no' more than three times to the first ten questions and 'yes' more than three times to the last ten questions, you should request extra guidance through your doctor or a specialised organisation for child and family care. Make sure you yourself are feeling good about yourself again, by processing your distressing birth or old hurts from your past with the help of a therapist. Sometimes you only realise what you lacked from your own parents (even if they withheld it without being aware of it) when you become a parent yourself. Your parents did their best; they too are the product of their own upbringing. The technical term for this is trans-generational trauma transmission. You are, as it were, inflicted by the unhappiness of your parents and their parents. The psychosocial-emotional problems and traumas are thus passed on from generation to generation (see the section on epigenetics at the end of this chapter). If you didn't feel safe at home when you were a child and didn't feel like you could go to your parents with your problems, you might not have a safe bond yourself. This can also happen if your parents had psychological problems and were therefore too preoccupied with themselves to be emotionally involved with you and your development. In this case it can be extra difficult for you to build a strong attachment with your child. If this feels familiar to you or your partner, get extra guidance for bringing up your children – for their sake.

If it still isn't easy for you to make contact with your baby, or if this doesn't (yet) feel straightforward, you can strengthen your bond by dancing together or singing, massaging your baby, bathing or showering together with your baby, reading stories or playing together, even if you are feeling anxious or depressed. Singing to your baby can calm her down for twice as long as talking to her; singing helps babies regulate their emotions. By doing fun activities with your baby you will automatically make contact with her more. Even if it doesn't feel quite right at first, keep persevering! When you smile at your baby, you invite her to smile back at you. You can also build a bond with your baby by looking where she's pointing or by playing a clapping or peek-a-boo game together.

"The birth was harder than I had imagined. I joked that it was a 'failed experiment'. The only thing that did work was breastfeeding my daughter. It seemed like my body and my breasts knew what they were supposed to do, while I was still thinking about the birth. There was not much connecting me to my baby, but when I nursed her, things literally flowed smoothly. While I fed her she watched me with wide-open eyes. At first, I couldn't bear that and I looked away. Nevertheless, the hormones did their work. Slowly, a bond grew between us. It gave me a good feeling when I fed her, it was like compensation for the 'failed' delivery. Once I had processed the delivery, my 'homework' was to massage Laurie every other day and on the remaining days to bathe or shower with her: 'bathing together, bonding together'. Now Laurie is two years old and we still bathe together once a week. If I hadn't kept a diary of the first year, I wouldn't have believed that I had felt nothing for her. She's my everything." (Flora, 29 years old)

How do you comfort a crying baby?

Most babies start crying more often and for longer about two weeks after birth. By then you don't have help from nurses and doctors anymore and you find yourselves alone with your baby. It's probably the first time in your life that you are responsible for someone else 24/7, someone who is completely dependent on you. The only way a baby can express his discontent is by crying. He will cry to say he is hungry, needs a clean nappy, is trying to burp or is tired. Babies also cry because they would rather be with you than alone in a cot or because they have stomach cramps, are sick or in pain. At around six weeks old, babies will cry two to two and a half hours a day. After 12 to 16 weeks the worst of the crying period should be over. Then a baby will "only" cry one to one and half hours a day. For premature babies, you count the weeks from their due date.

3 x 3 x 3
Let your doctor know if your baby cries excessively: more than three hours a day, at least three days a week, for more than three weeks. She can rule out a physiological cause or refer you to a paediatrician. Even if your baby cries less than this but if you feel you can't take it anymore or if you are worried, discuss it with your doctor. In 95% (!) of cases, no physiological problem is diagnosed and "luckily" it's a healthy baby who "communicates" by crying. Babies that cry a lot cannot easily comfort themselves and unfortunately are not easily comforted by their parents either. It might give you peace of mind if a doctor is able to rule out a medical or physical reason for the crying.

Babies that cry a lot often have short and restless sleeps. Their flailing arms (due to the startle or Moro reflex) wake them up and they begin to cry. Because of this they don't fall into a sleeping rhythm, they're tired and have less energy to feed properly. Often, babies who don't sleep well drink voraciously, making them choke and bring up their milk. This means they don't have enough food to digest. In addition they can over-stretch, lifting their back from the ground they are lying on. They will often develop a preferred lying position, leading to a flattened skull on one side. All these reasons can explain increased crying.

A baby's crying is heart-wrenching and nerve-wracking for new parents, who might feel like their nerves are laid exposed on the surface of their skin. The baby's cries cause electric-like impulses, similar to when you knock your funny bone in your elbow. When your nerves are already raw because of a distressing birth experience, you are far less able to handle things than before. You want to do everything you can to help your baby but nothing seems to work. People around you offer well-intentioned advice that often only adds to your frustration. It seems like everyone thinks they know what is best for your child, but these advisors aren't cooped up for hours at a time with a crying baby. When your baby starts to cry again, you switch on your alert, over-sensitive mode again and your baby's cries go right through to your bones.

Crying babies form the greatest pressure (on relationships) in the first months after birth! It's normal that you take the tension and frustration out on the person closest to you: your partner. You just need each other so much as parents and you are both so tired, that you really don't need this extra irritation. There might also be feelings of guilt towards your baby. It's only human to be (extremely) annoyed now and then at your baby's constant crying. I have purposely written "to be annoyed at your baby's constant crying", not to be confused with being annoyed at your baby itself. The constant crying makes you crazy, not the baby, who can't help itself. So if you (very understandably) are annoyed by the crying, it doesn't mean you are annoyed by your baby. If you can separate your baby from the crying, most parents find it easier to "survive". Luckily, there are a number of remedies that work wonders on most babies. First of all, it can help to carry your baby close to your body as much as possible (kangaroo care). You can use a special sling or baby carrier for this. The baby rocks back and forth, just as he did when he was still inside your body. Bodily contact leads to reduced crying.

Babies who are carried ten hours a day cry 50% less. The average Western baby has about six hours a day of physical contact (between feeding, changing, cuddling, bathing and carrying). I often tell my clients that babies are "skin hungry". Touching and skin-on-skin contact reduce feelings of stress and normalise the heart rate and breathing in babies up to two years old. The less stress babies have, the better their brains can develop. Eighty per cent of brain development takes place in the first year. Research on rats shows that young rats that have a lot of physical contact with their mother build a social buffer against stress. Putting a baby in the bath just before their crying time begins is another good tip. Most babies sleep more peacefully if they have had a bath just before. After the bath you can massage your baby if he is still calm (see more on baby massage on page 109).

The Karp method

American paediatrician Harvey Karp suggests that human babies are born three months earlier than they should be and are therefore immature compared to other animals. It isn't possible to leave the baby in the uterus for three extra months – it would then grow too big for a vaginal birth. However, a good way to comfort a baby in the first three months is to recreate the conditions of the womb as closely as possible. Imagine you are your baby: in the womb he heard and felt you (his mother) constantly around him. If he's then laid alone in a bed for 20 hours a day, it's a brutal transition. In his book *The Happiest Baby on the Block*, Dr. Karp sets out a technique to calm a baby in five steps. Many of my clients have tried these steps and are happy with the result.

It's important to carry out the steps as precisely as possible, as they are set out below. In his book, Dr. Karp compares this to the knee-reflex. If a doctor taps your knee at exactly the right spot, your lower leg flies up as a reflex. If she taps just an inch away from the spot, nothing happens. This is the same for the calming reflex. It doesn't work if you try a bit of one step and a modified version of another. You can, however, see which step works best for your baby. Some babies are more sensitive to sound and so take most easily to the third step. Others might be calmed by movement, making the fourth step the most appropriate. As first, all five steps are necessary, especially for babies who cry very loudly. When your baby's crying starts to subside and becomes calmer, you can eliminate one step. Dr. Karp calls it the Five S's technique (swaddling, side or stomach position, shushing, swinging, sucking), which activates the calming reflex so the crying stops, as if you've found the "off button".

Step 1: Swaddling
To swaddle your baby you need a piece of stretchable cotton or woollen cloth, of at least one square metre.
a)   Lay the cloth out in a diamond shape in front of you and fold down the upper corner.
b)   Lay the baby down on the cloth with his head off the cloth, and his shoulders on the cloth.
c)   Take the left side and fold it across his right arm – which is along his side – and tuck it quite firmly under your baby's back.
d)   Pick up the lower corner and fold it upwards over your baby's left shoulder.
e)   Wrap the remaining right corner over the bay's left arm up to his chest and fold it inwards.
f)   Fold the remaining fabric around his back and around to his chest.

Don't swaddle if your baby:
- Has a fever;
- Is sick or has a bad cold;
- Has (untreated) eczema;
- Has had a vaccination in the past 24 hours;
- Has hip dysplasia;
- Was in a breech position for a long time during your pregnancy.

If in doubt, ask your doctor or midwife.

Unsuitable materials for swaddling:
- Fleece blankets;
- Blankets;
- Flannel cloths;
- Synthetic fabrics;
- Quilts or duvets.

These materials are all too warm. Your baby isn't yet able to let you know when he is too warm, let alone kick off his blankets. Overheating in babies is a real danger.

If you find it too complicated to swaddle your baby, you can buy ready-made swaddling "blankets"/wraps. Swaddling gives your baby the same "constricted" feeling he had in the womb. As mentioned above, your baby can feel lost on his own in a (big) cot. It's important for babies to have the space and time to develop physically when they aren't swaddled. Schedule "playtimes" between feeds and naps in which your baby can move freely. Even when your baby is swaddled he needs to have sufficient room around his hips to be able to stretch and lift his legs. Your baby will enjoy it even more if you "talk" to him during these playtimes, for example, by sticking your tongue out slowly or holding your hand in a fist 30 centimetres from his eyes and slowly opening and closing your hand. You will notice that your baby imitates these movements. Obviously a baby who is only a couple of weeks old isn't able to lift his fist up and open his hand in front of his chest, but if you watch his hand carefully you will see a movement. After changing your baby you can lay him on his tummy on his changing mat, while always watching him carefully. This is good for developing his motor skills. From four months onwards you should start reducing the swaddling. From that age, babies can roll over and a swaddled baby who rolls on to his tummy is at a higher risk of cot death.

Step 2: Side or stomach position

A baby lying on his back can startle himself awake by waving his arms as a result of his Moro reflex. This reflex won't affect him if he's sleeping on his side or front. You can lay a swaddled baby on his side with his tummy resting on your lower arm (your left arm if you're right-handed and vice versa). In this way your baby is "hanging" on your arm. For extra support and security, you can hold his back against your body. This position is also called the reverse breastfeeding position. This "hanging" position reminds the baby of his time in the womb where, after all, he never lay flat on his back. The warm pressure of your lower arm on his stomach helps to soothe stomach cramps or wind. Your baby is held close to your body and can hear your heart beating. This is a familiar and trusted sound for him because he heard it constantly while he was inside. Once he has fallen asleep you can lay him swaddled and on his back in his cot.

Step 3: Shushing

Babies are able to hear from 28 weeks of gestation and they are exposed to continuous noise in your body. There are noises from your intestines, your blood circulation and from the outside world. In terms of intensity, the sound of your blood circulating is equivalent to that of a vacuum cleaner. Intuitively, many parents try to put their children to sleep by driving a car, turning on a hair dryer or actually vacuuming. Parents all over the world make more or less the same sound to calm a crying baby: ssshhh. You can buy special devices, CDs and DVDs that imitate the sounds of the womb: the so-called "white noise". You can imitate the sound of blood circulation yourself: make a ssshhh sound about five centimetres from your baby's ear, just slightly louder than the baby is crying. When he was in your womb, your baby heard your blood stream louder than anything else (85 decibels!). If he can hear his own crying (80 decibels) louder than your shushing, it won't be effective. This might take some getting used to for you. It might make you feel like a strict schoolteacher who wants to silence a classroom of children. But for your baby, this is the closest to the sound of your blood circulating and it works surprisingly well. You see and feel your baby relaxing. The louder he cries, the louder you shush. Try to make it deeper in your throat – more "shh" than a hard hissing "sss".

Step 4: Swinging

When your baby was still inside your womb, you rocked him to and fro all day long with your movements: a wonderful kind of wave pool or rocking crib. This is why most babies start rocking themselves in utero when their mothers sit or lie down. They try to create their own wave pool. Once they are born they can't create that movement anymore. The wave pool stops. When they move it's usually just waving their arms and legs, which often startles them. Thus moving doesn't necessarily calm them down. However, if you move around while holding them the effect is much more like the way they were rocked by your body when you were pregnant, which evokes pleasant memories for them. You will notice yourself which movements are most pleasing to your baby: from side to side or up and down. It's a question of trial and error and patient practice. Ask your doctor or paediatric centre the best way to move with your child or on your arm if you're still unsure.

In any case, ensure that you NEVER shake your baby hard. His neck isn't yet strong enough and his head therefore wobbles around more than the head of an adult or a child. Hard shaking can lead to Shaken Baby Syndrome (SBS). In Holland and Flanders almost 50 babies a year are hospitalised for a brain haemorrhage or injury and about four babies die because of SBS. If your baby's crying is driving you mad, lay him in his cot and walk out of the room until you have calmed down yourself. If you're worried that you can't control yourself (anymore), call somebody and ask them to come over and help you.

Step 5: Sucking

This fifth step is so natural that you have probably already done it by yourself. Every baby has a sucking instinct – it's how he comforts himself. It doesn't matter if your baby is breast- or bottle-fed. It doesn't really matter either what he sucks on, as long as he can suck. If you are breastfeeding, it's advisable to not give your baby a dummy in the first few weeks, so that he doesn't develop nipple confusion. If your baby is bottle-fed you can give her a dummy. Most babies need time to get used to the dummy. You can also let your baby suck on your thumb or little finger. When you put your little finger in the baby's mouth you can feel when the baby stops sucking. You can sometimes feel her tongue pushing in a different way against your finger but because you automatically apply counter-pressure, your baby isn't able to push your finger out of her mouth. A dummy doesn't push back, so when the baby stops sucking or pushes against it with her tongue, it will simply fall out of her mouth. You can help your baby by training the sucking reflex a little. Pull softly on the dummy or pull your finger back a little. Most babies will then suck harder and after some practice will manage to keep the dummy in their mouth.

The four-minute-method

For babies older than six months, there is another method that can help: the four-minute-method. Try this method if you are sure your baby doesn't have a fever, is not sick or hungry and doesn't have a dirty nappy. It's important that both parents stand behind it and that you don't give up once you've started. Check the cot is at the right temperature. Establish an evening routine, perhaps with a bath, a massage with oil and a lullaby. Put your baby in the cot and sing the lullaby again. Then walk away (still singing softly, if you like) and let your baby cry for four minutes. It helps to set a timer (on your phone) to keep track because four minutes can seem like an eternity when your baby is crying. After the four minutes, go back to your child and talk or sing to him until he is calm again. You can also gently put your hand on his head or his stomach. Then walk away and let him cry again for four minutes. It can help if both parents alternate being "on duty". The parent "on duty" applies the method while the other parent tries to sleep through the crying using ear plugs. The following night the other parent takes over. If one of you finds it particularly hard to let your baby cry and your partner can manage it better, then perhaps the parent who finds it less difficult can do two or three nights in a row, perhaps at the weekend.

Co-sleeping

In non-Western cultures, parents and children often sleep in the same room ("rooming-in") and nursing mothers often sleep in the same bed as their baby. However, in some cultures there's an ongoing debate about the risks associated with co-sleeping for babies younger than six months. You can now buy special, half-open cots called co-sleepers that can be attached to the parents' bed so your baby is protected but still close to you. You can also place the cot next to your own bed (rooming-in).

Baby massage

Baby massage can help babies to feel comfortable. Your baby relaxes from the massage and you relax when you massage him. Most importantly, massage can strengthen the interaction and thus the bond between you. You can join a baby massage class with other parents and their babies, take private lessons or buy a DVD that explains the technique step by step.

Extra guidance at home

Speak to your doctor about the possibility of receiving extra guidance, for example, through video-interaction training in your home. In this training, a prevention worker comes to your house and films the interaction between you and your baby. Together you observe how your baby reacts to your voice and how the baby tries to make contact with you. Once you learn to recognise the signals from your baby, your (self-)confidence will grow as will your baby's confidence in himself and in you. Very soon you will both be in a positive growth spiral. Parent-baby video-interaction training is advisable for parents with psychiatric disorders. Trauma, PTSD, postnatal depression and anxiety disorder come under this category, even though they are usually of a temporary nature. Don't hesitate to ask for help, for the sake of your child, to prevent the situation from getting worse. The sooner you address it, the sooner you can break the negative spiral. It also helps to write down at the end of each day what went well, if you made contact or had fun with your baby, or to take a photo every day of a precious moment (see the end of Chapter 3).

"I was terribly nervous about them coming to my house to film me. To be honest I was afraid they would take my child away from me. Fortunately, it was always the same lady who came – she was like a sort of grandmother for me. She made the videos and after a while I forgot she was there. She never once said something bad about the way I behaved with my son. She pointed out when he was looking for my attention and how I could react to that. After a few sessions she showed me the difference between the first time she filmed us and the most recent videos. I became very emotional when I saw how much I had grown as a mother." (Sophie, 25 years old)

For those who want to delve deeper: epigenetics

The following is quite a technical and scientific account.
I'm including this for medical professionals and others who may be interested, because this field of research is one of the reasons I wrote this book. The impact of PTSD complaints goes further than you might expect at first sight. You can skip this paragraph as long as you remember that it's important to do something about your PTSD complaints, for your own sake and for the sake of your future children.

Professor Rachel Yehuda collected data in New York from a group of pregnant women who lived or worked close to the Twin Towers at the time of the attacks of September 11 2001. Approximately half of the women in the research group were diagnosed with Post-Traumatic Stress Disorder (PTSD). All the women with PTSD had less cortisol in their saliva than those who hadn't developed PTSD. Cortisol is a stress hormone. It increases the sugar (glucose) in your blood to prepare you for fight or flight in stressful situations. Cortisol is produced by your adrenal glands. If you have been exposed to stress for a long stretch of time, for example, due to a burnout or untreated PTSD, your adrenal glands become exhausted and your body is incapable of producing sufficient cortisol. This means you can't react adequately to stress or to new stressful situations. You become unbalanced more easily and tolerate much less. You have symptoms similar to those of a burnout.

The babies of the women who were in their third trimester (six to nine months pregnant) at the time of the attacks from which they developed PTSD all (!) had less cortisol in their saliva and were less able to deal with stress or stressful situations. This was not only the case just after they were born: ten years on, those children still showed the same traits. It's possible that PTSD causes a change in the genes of a mother or pregnant woman and it seems she can pass this on to her children. PTSD alters the body's response to stress, i.e. the way the body deals with stress. The hypothalamic-pituitary-adrenal axis (HPA axis or HTPA axis) plays an important role in human stress responses. The HPA axis seems to be permanently changed in the children of women who had PTSD when they were pregnant. Since it takes a long time for generations to reproduce (minimum 20 years, on average 29 years) it will be a long time before we can make solid statements about this. Research with rats (whose generations reproduce much faster) show that changes in the HPA axis are hereditary, but whether this also applies to humans is still unclear.

The field of research is called epigenetics. Epigenetics explores to what extent we can turn our genes "on" or "off". In the past we believed that only nature and nurture determined a child's development. Yehuda and her colleagues recently showed that the expression of all of 16 genes is different in people who developed PTSD following the events of 9/11, compared with people who also experienced the same events but didn't develop PTSD. The genetic profile of these women was unknown before the attacks, therefore it can't be proved that the change in gene expression is caused by PTSD.

Research with rats shows that the altered gene expression (if a gene is switched "on" or "off") is passed on to descendants. In the Netherlands, Professor Tessa Roseboom did doctoral research into the health of babies born in the Wilhelmina hospital in Amsterdam during the Dutch famine (the winter of 1944–45). Her research shows that undernourishment in mothers during their pregnancy had permanent consequences on the health of the child later in life, even after that child reached adulthood. Prof. Roseboom used a useful metaphor during her talk to explain epigenetics: she compared it to the mixing equipment used by a DJ. Humans come about from the merging of an egg cell (from a woman) and a sperm cell (from a man). Both these cells contain a genetic code. At first, the fertilised egg divides itself extremely fast into 2-4-8-16-32-64-128... etc. identical cells. These cells therefore have the same genetic code. As the embryo develops further, different cells perform different functions in different parts of the body. The cells differentiate themselves and specialise. Some cells can contract rhythmically (such as in the heart), while others discern and pass on light (in the eye). This happens because a certain gene in one particular cell is "switched on" while another gene is "switched off". In other cells, that would be the other way around. A whole new human is "mixed" out of the DNA of her parents, as if by a DJ with a mixer. Just as a DJ's mixer has many volume buttons to determine how loud each song is played, the DNA has similar "volume buttons", which determine to what extent a cell performs a certain function. For example, in one cell, the volume can be turned up to maximum, causing that cell to produce a large amount of a protein that makes it possible to rhythmically contract (such as cells in the heart), while that exact same DNA is switched off in another cell, so that cell cannot produce the protein responsible for contracting. In the latter cell, a different button is on maximum because its function is different. When somebody experiences an event as traumatic, the volume of certain parts of the DNA can change, thus changing the function of the cells. The DNA itself doesn't change, but the volume determines whether a certain melody is heard or not.

You can imagine that an anxious pregnant woman produces large amounts of stress hormones. The baby does that too and is prepared – through its mother – for a stressful existence outside the womb. That baby will react more intensely and will be more nervous than a baby that grew in a stress-free womb. For this reason, I also guide women in processing previous birth experiences during their pregnancy, in order to ensure that the volume buttons on the DNA mixer are in the best possible position for the new baby.

Petra's

STORY

I was looking forward to giving birth. I felt well prepared:
I had taken a pregnancy course and had made a birth plan
together with my partner. I was going to deliver my baby at
home in the bath. At around 36 weeks my waters broke – just
a little too early to be allowed a home birth. The baby's head
was also not properly engaged. We had to go to the hospital.
I wanted to have as natural a birth as possible, preferably
without pain medication. Because I needed a drip to make the
contractions stronger, the gynaecologist advised me to have
an epidural. How was I to know that I wouldn't have any feeling
in my legs? I lay there, feeling like a ladybird that was on its
back, fighting in vain to turn itself over.

The ward was busy but I was lucky to have a very kind
nurse. She explained everything to me and apologised every
time she had to increase the dose of medication to strengthen
my contractions. After a couple of hours I began to shake and
had a fever. The baby's heartbeat also rose. They decided to go
for a C-section – or wait, have another look – no C-section. It
seemed as though no one was prepared to make the decision.
Peter was eventually born with the help of the ventouse. They
laid him on my belly and I felt very happy; happy that it was
over and happy that Peter was doing so well. Suddenly I felt
blood streaming between my legs. I nearly fainted. Someone
pressed on my stomach and pulled on the umbilical cord,
which broke off. They shoved the baby into my husband's arms
and rushed me topsy-turvy into an operating room. I will never
forget the look in my husband's eyes. I thought I was going to die
and I could see that he thought so too. I don't remember anything
of the operation, or from the time after it. It took about three
months before I had physically recovered from the birth.

My son Peter cried a lot. Whenever he began to cry, his cries went right through me and I reacted by putting a bottle of milk in his mouth. Eventually he was admitted to hospital under observation because of excessive crying. In the hospital he cried much less, so we were sent home, where he began to cry again almost immediately. We went back to the hospital and he was finally diagnosed with silent reflux. I was a wreck. I sometimes got angry with Peter. Before he arrived on the scene my life had been great. Within a year of his arrival everything was a mess. I was so preoccupied with Peter that I had no time for my husband or for myself. I decided to cut off my long hair – with hindsight that was a sign that I wasn't well. I really felt traumatised by Peter's constant crying. I once put him in the garden shed because I could still hear his screeches through my ear plugs. The only thing that seemed to help was to feed him. The doctor told me to give him less food as he was already overweight. I didn't tell them I sometimes gave him twice the recommended number of bottles in one day. I thinned it down a little with water, but still... Peter smiled at other people, but never at me. I didn't smile at him anymore either. I looked after him and we tolerated each other.

After a year and a half, I was unexpectedly pregnant with our second child. I was afraid and sought extra guidance from a coach. With my coach, I was first able to admit that I didn't feel a bond with Peter and that I didn't dare give birth again. We started the work of processing the distressing birth experience. This helped to calm me and it also seemed to calm him. The gynaecologist suggested that a planned C-section might help me to be less tense during my pregnancy. That took a weight off my shoulders.

A brighter period was underway. I had no pregnancy complaints and things were going okay with Peter. He threw tantrums, but which two-year-old doesn't? I gained confidence in the pregnancy and made preparations for the birth. Strangely, once I knew I would have a C-section I felt I was being taken seriously by the doctors and I was able to consider having a normal delivery. The C-section was due to take place two days before my due date. A week before that I began to have contractions. The baby's head was fully engaged and we agreed with the gynaecologist to wait and see how my labour went. Within a couple of hours Nina was lying on my stomach. What a difference there had been between the two births! Just a couple of hours later I was allowed to go home.

Nina was an exemplary baby. It felt easy and natural to care for her. Unfortunately Peter was very jealous. He had become a highly strung, overweight three-year-old. At school he pushed other children around and demanded one-on-one attention from the teacher. She told me Peter needed to learn frustration tolerance and advised me to sign him up for play therapy. I decided to go back to my coach. During some very painful sessions I realised that although he wasn't lacking anything in terms of physical care, he could probably feel my rejection of him in spite of the care. This came from the distressing start we had had together. We both still bore scars from the birth and the year that followed it.

I taught Peter to manage his emotions, instead of stuffing food into his mouth every time he got angry. Before I had been "numbing" his emotions by feeding him whenever he was angry, frustrated or sad. His crying pushed my "bad-mother-button". I also resented him for making me feel like a bad mother. He felt that deep inside and that made him hang on to me; we both ended up trapped in a negative spiral.

I also learned to manage my own emotions and thoughts. It wasn't Peter who was unbearable, but the things he did were sometimes unbearable. I wasn't a bad mother, but my behaviour reinforced Peter's negative behaviour. Slowly I learned to trust that I was doing the best I could and that this was good enough. By the time Peter finally started play therapy, things were going much better with us. You should see him today: the sweetest child in the class. You should see me today: the nicest mum at the school gate, complete with high heels and long hair!

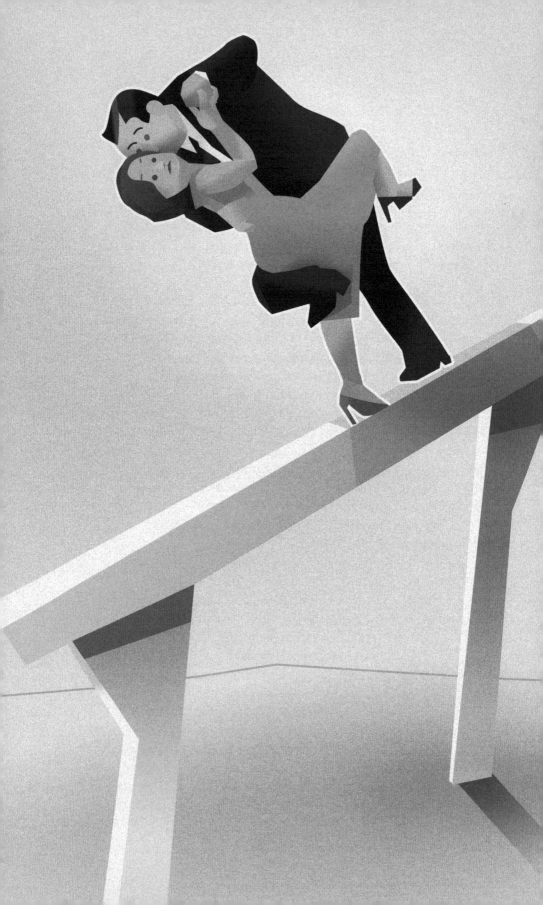

CHAPTER 5

A distressing birth – how it affects your relationship

A distressing or traumatic birth doesn't only leave its mark on you and your baby. It can also put pressure on your relationship with your partner. One in five parents – mothers as well as fathers – have adjustment problems, in any case, in the first year after a baby arrives. The symptoms associated with these adjustment problems are similar to those of a mild depression. It's completely normal to experience small problems in a new life situation. Unfortunately, it's hardly ever talked about, and this leaves many parents thinking that they are the only ones to encounter these problems.

There is life before children and life with children. One of the most common stumbling blocks is that in a life with children you simply have very little time for each other. On average, new parents talk to each other just five to seven minutes a day. Their time is taken over by practical worries. When they talk to each other, it's mainly about logistics: who's picking up the kids today and who's doing the grocery shopping.

For many couples, the busy period following the birth of their (first) child is the first time their relationship is under strain. Add to that lack of sleep, insecurity, worry about the baby and hormonal see-sawing, and before you know it you're taking your stress out on each other. This is even more pertinent if one or both partners experienced the birth as a traumatic event. Different people process traumatic events in different ways (see Chapter 2). It's tough to undergo a difficult birth when you're the woman in labour, but it's also tough to watch your partner suffer through the birth while you stand by, pretty much powerless to do anything.

"It was as if I ceased to matter since Ella was born. Our daughter took places one to ten in my wife's life and, oh yes… there was also a man in the house somewhere who used to be her life partner. I felt excluded by her so I focused instead on my work. At least at the office I felt valued and appreciated. It sounds childish when I read this, but that was a very lonely time for me. I missed my wife and didn't know how to reach her. She didn't want to do anything fun just with me; the baby had to come with us everywhere. She went to bed early in the evenings and, because she was breastfeeding, I didn't feel like there was very much I could contribute. We had tried to have sex one time since the birth, but it was so painful for Rita that I didn't dare mention it again. That made me even lonelier. It's a huge cliché, but during a conference overseas, I slept with a colleague. After an eight-year-long monogamous relationship! I confessed my infidelity to Rita and we started going to couple therapy. The weird part was to discover during the therapy sessions that Rita had also felt lonely in the first year after Ella was born." (Bram, 31 years old)

"During the birth I was afraid Ella was going to die. Several times the umbilical cord was around her neck and she needed extra oxygen once she was born. It was very alarming for me. Being a mother makes you so vulnerable because you love your child so much. I was overflowing with love… and with worry for Ella. I was constantly occupied with her, checked several times a night that she was breathing and kept her as close as possible to me during the day. I hated having to go back to work. My office moved to another city and there was a reorganization that allowed me to opt for redundancy with six months' pay. I jumped at the opportunity. Before Ella I would have discussed it extensively with Bram first, but this time I just informed him of my decision. I didn't want to do anything but stay at home with Ella but, to be honest, I also found it hard to suddenly be a stay-at-home mum. Bram's life went on as usual, while my life had changed in every way. When I heard he had cheated on me with his colleague, I felt betrayed.

With hindsight, I understand how it could have happened. Since Ella was born we had been living parallel lives. His infidelity was a wake-up call for me, for Bram and for our relationship. It cost us many tears and many therapy sessions but we made it through together.

I also had a number of sessions on my own, to help me process the trauma of the birth. The birth influenced my behaviour that first year to a great extent. I was so afraid of losing Ella that I was constantly trying to control everything and was hyper-vigilant. There was simply no room in my head for Bram. Whenever he wanted to talk about his work or anything else, I couldn't concentrate on what he was saying. Luckily, we are now back to being a real couple as well as parenting Ella together. I have a lovely new part-time job and Bram is working one day less. We've found a new balance." (Rita, 26 years old)

> Your partner might also be a great disappointment to you during the birth. You think you know each other through and through, but during childbirth you might discover traits in your partner that you would rather not have seen. You had expected/hoped/thought that your partner would support you and actively coach you; that he would speak up for you and protect your interests like a lion when you couldn't do it yourself because of the pain or the contractions, but in reality you felt let down by him. Perhaps he made silly jokes because he was so nervous, or maybe he watched television instead of massaging your aching back.
>
> Your partner can also have been disappointed in your conduct during the birth: how you dealt with the pain, how you let yourself go, how you excluded him, while he had hoped you would birth the baby "together".

"Harry was such a disappointment to me during and just after the birth. It was a serious blow to our relationship. We had agreed in advance that he would look after me, that we would take on the contractions together – just as we had practised together during the antenatal classes – and that he would stand up for me if I wasn't able to. But then, when the contractions began, he wanted to sleep a bit more. He hardly breathed together with me – he left that to the nurse to do – while he played with his phone. And he didn't stand up for me at all during the whole experience, which lasted 24 hours. In the week after the birth he fell ill with the flu. The visiting nurse spent more time looking after him than after me. I thought he was really a wimp.

Looking back, I realise it was at that moment that I decided I didn't need him anymore. I behaved like a single mother with a roommate. If he sought closeness, wanted to do something fun together or wanted to take Bob out alone, I had other plans. My life was filled up with work, with Bob, my friends and my family but I had no time or attention to give to Harry. It was as if I wanted to punish him for his behaviour during the birth. I realised this, for the first time, during the couple therapy sessions, and later – with difficulty – managed to express my disappointment. That gave Harry the chance to express his own disappointment with my 'unreachability'. We really wouldn't have been able to express this without a neutral third person; we would instead have attacked each other. For me it was difficult to accept that my tendency to withdraw could be explained by my parents' divorce. Because I hadn't wanted to choose a side back then, I went to live by myself. With hindsight, I was much too young for that, but back then I felt I had chosen a stance of independence – of 'I don't need anybody'. I had initially felt safe with Harry, but because he hadn't been there for me while I was in labour and the week after I gave birth, I withdrew back into my 'it doesn't matter what you do to me, I can manage alone' attitude. I see now that he really had tried to reach me but I didn't let him close." (Eve, 24 years old)

"I didn't recognise Eve at all during the birth. She had always been so strong and independent and suddenly she was so needy, lying there in pain and moaning very loudly. It made me nervous and giggly at the same time. I tried making jokes, hoping it would make her laugh but it seemed like she had pushed out her sense of humour along with the baby. The week after that I came down with a bad flu, so I spent the week mostly in the guest room because I didn't want to infect Eve and Bob. Every time I wanted to do something fun there was always a reason why it wasn't convenient. If I spent a day home alone with Bob, there was always something I had done wrong. Before the birth we almost never fought, but now we were sometimes like two cockerels screaming at each other. It drove me mad when Eve shut herself off from me. She behaved like an ice queen and I was her subject. It was an eye-opener when I heard how lonely she had felt during the birth and afterwards when I was sick; how disappointed she had been in me. I also learned that our clashes often sprang from the fact that she (supposedly) didn't need anybody and I really needed to be needed. But because I was afraid of the whole childbirth experience, I made silly jokes to cover my fear and that was the start of the annoyance and disconnection between us. It was very useful to have a neutral translator/judge in the room when we talked. We had to learn to take a time-out in order to cool down and then to talk calmly about what had happened, why the situation escalated and what we both needed. Neither of us had learned from our parents to talk about things like that." (Harry, 26 years old)

You can learn to communicate – the four-part Nonviolent Communication process

When you become parents, in addition to being partners, you acquire a new, all-encompassing role in your life, next to all the other roles you already fulfil (being a child, brother/sister, friend, colleague, sports partner...). Unfortunately, you aren't given more hours in the day in which to fulfil this new role. For this reason it's very important to keep communicating using the following process, which is based on Marshall Rosenberg's theory of *Nonviolent Communication*.

1. **Observation:** What exactly do you see or hear: Use the "I" sentences rather than "you" sentences. The other person can view "you" sentences as attacks, which will make them want to counter-attack, and the discussion will escalate before you know it.
2. **Feelings:** How do you feel? Take a moment to identify the emotions flowing through you. This will make it easier to put them into words. It will also make it easier for the other person to understand how you feel and why. Sometimes people can "press your buttons" without realising: they say something that touches a raw spot and it makes you react more violently than you intended.

3. **Needs:** What do you need? What does your partner need? If you expect that your partner knows exactly what your needs are and will fulfil your unexpressed needs, I can guarantee you'll be disappointed.

4. **Requests:** What do you mean and what does your partner mean? Do the words you use really express the meaning you want to convey? Is there anything that needs to be made clearer in terms of meaning? What would you like to achieve with this discussion?

I like to use the example of loading the dishwasher. When you ask your partner to load the dishwasher, there's a strong chance he will say *"yes"*. You just haven't asked when he's going to do it. As far as he's concerned, it can be in the evening or the following morning, but you expect him to do it straight away, because that's what you would do. You are looking at the situation from your own standpoint and you expect him to react as you would. Except that he is not you. If he carries on reading the newspaper, you can start to feel irritated. *"I'll just do it myself."* You noisily and angrily load the dishwasher. Your partner is unaware of any animosity. He had intended to do it, just not right now. Why are you so upset? He has no idea... Why don't you let him do it his way? Why are you always complaining ever since you had children? No idea...

"Our twins, Jodie and Doug, were born premature. We started having problems when Marceline went back to work. We both have enjoyable and challenging jobs and neither of us wanted to give them up. We had decided that we would both keep working full-time (36 hours a week), spread over four days of nine hours. That would give us each a day at home with the twins and they would only have to spend three days at the crèche. It sounded like a good plan, but we hadn't taken into account the health issues that premature babies encounter: they were often sick, Doug needed physiotherapy, Jodie had hearing problems and needed a whole host of tests. We were both working very hard to keep all the balls in the air. Marceline, who had been hard-hit by the birth, found it hard to concentrate and was very anxious and over-protective. We were both overstretched and we took it out on each other.

Our weekend plans were also divergent. I wanted to sleep late and rest at home, while Marceline wanted to have 'fun family time' and invite friends over for dinner. This was hard because the children needed a lot of rest and routine, much more than we did. Just as we had everything ready and were out the door, it was time to go back home for a nap. When friends came over, one of us would be in the kitchen while the other was busy with the twins. Our relationship was crumbling before our eyes and we had no idea how to turn it around. We blamed each other that it wasn't 'fun' at home anymore. We didn't have time for anything: sports or an evening out with friends. We were just rushing about all the time... And arguing, all evening, sometimes deep into the night, just when we needed our sleep so badly.

Marceline started seeing a coach in order to process the birth experience. After a couple of sessions she started to feel better. After that we went to the coach together to talk about our relationship. It was enlightening to see how we resented each other for how complicated our lives had become since the twins. By focusing on what was happening between us, we both felt less personally attacked. We understood what was going on, what provoked our arguments and how we could prevent escalation. The first time we used a time-out and came back to the discussion once we had calmed down was a turning point for us.

We began looking for practical solutions to take the pressure off. The paediatrician preferred us not to send our babies to the crèche because of the increased exposure to infection. Instead we got a wonderful nanny, Jane, whose arrival brought peace back to our family. We both took a day off per week as parental leave. This gave us the chance to do other things, such as sports, and it took the pressure off weekends, which are also less hectic. What struck us during the therapy sessions was how we knew exactly how to rub each other's 'raw spots' from our pasts. For example, I couldn't deal with the fact that Marceline had psychological issues because I grew up with a mother who had psychological issues. It therefore made me shut myself off from Marceline just when she needed me most to be present and supportive. She, on the other hand, complained too much (in my view) about trivial things and it turned out she did this in order to involve me more in family life. We also discovered that we provoked and hurt each other just to get a reaction, out of fear that we would lose each other. We hadn't realised that on our own. Instead of hurting each other, we learned to just say what we needed. Usually that was something very simple: understanding, a listening ear, a hug, time alone. By expressing our needs and by treating each other as a 'best friend' instead of a critical partner we became much nicer and more tolerant towards each other. We made it through the storm together." (Steve, 33 years old)

Growing up in a warm and close nest

Growing up in a loving and harmonious household offers a child some protection against emotional, psychological and social problems later in life. A strong relationship between his/her parents is the basis. Unfortunately, many relationships turn sour; more than two-thirds of couples who are currently expecting their first child will have separated by the time their child is four years old. This means that an increasing number of children grow up in single-parent or blended families. Children are extremely receptive to tension between their parents. They feel happier and safer with parents who are "happily" divorced – parents who speak in a neutral or positive way about each other, who acknowledge each other as co-parents and who bring up the children together – than with parents who live in the same house but fight all the time.

I wish for all children that their parents invest in maintaining their relationship, for example, by calling on the help of a therapist in time, preferably before the relationship is damaged beyond repair. You don't need to have an ailing relationship to see a therapist. You can also choose to go to one in order to invest in a healthy relationship that can be made even better and to strengthen the bond between you with the help of a coach.

In my practice I use *Emotionally Focused Therapy* (EFT), which was developed by psychologist Sue Johnson (known for her bestseller *Hold Me Tight*). What makes this different from other forms of couple therapy is that the "patient" is the problematic interaction between the partners, rather than the partners themselves. The interaction is "the enemy", not the man or woman. Together you battle this enemy, instead of battling each other.

EFT couple therapy has a 70% effectiveness rate, almost twice as high as other forms of couple therapy. I always hope that parents come to me before the situation and the relationship have completely escalated. Building and propping up is easier than rebuilding on wreckage, where first the debris needs to be cleared before a new stable base can be created.

EFT examines the picture you have of yourself and your partner and the experiences you may have had in previous love relationships as well as your relationship with your parents. Next, it looks at all the things that are going well, the strong points of the relationship, and where the problems or grievances are. Both parents fill in a questionnaire (separately) and read their answers to each other during a session. Expressing needs can be particularly enlightening. You often assume that your partner can guess your needs or that he/she doesn't care, but how can they fill a need that you don't express? Perhaps you'd like your partner to listen to you without trying to find solutions and giving you advice, and he/she thinks that he/she is helping you by offering solutions to your problems. This exercise can probably help you talk to each other in a different way and allow you to see the stumbling blocks in your relationship and also your unfulfilled needs.

Assignment:
Describe – separately – the story of your love

- How and where did you meet?
- What was the first stage (of being in love) like?
- Can you pinpoint a specific event or period that marks the start of the problems or irritations between you?
- Have you had problems before? If so, how did you deal with them and how did you get out of them?
- What ideas about love did you receive from your parents? (or from your parents' divorce?)
- What ideas about love have you retained from your previous love relationships? (or from a previous divorce?)
- What are the strong points in your relationship?
- What could be improved in your relationship?
- Briefly describe the problem with your relationship:
    - What is your part of the problem?
    - What is your partner's part of the problem?
    - What do you think a solution might be?
- What do you need most from your partner right now? (Circle or insert your own words)

comfort	attention	recognition
respect	to be seen	to feel you've been heard
to feel wanted	touch	to be held
hugs	sex	reassurance
safety	to be needed	closeness
approval	acceptance	to feel you're strong together
to be accepted as you are	understanding	freedom
to be "important" to him/her	independence	to feel loved
appreciation	compliments	trust
fairness	sharing feelings	vulnerability
harmony (as opposed to conflict)	doing fun things together	support
sharing household tasks more fairly	listening	security
care	free time/"me-time"	rest/silence
humour	clarity	structure
relaxation	a fresh start	sharing responsibility
intimacy	feeling good together	friendship
help/support	connection	solidarity/complicity
protection	time for hobbies/sports	....
....	....	....

The more comprehensively you answer the questions, and the more clearly you illustrate your needs with examples, the greater the chance you will get a "connecting" discussion moving. A connecting discussion is one in which both partners feel they are being heard, understood, recognised, known, seen, respected and accepted. You both know you are worth the effort and important to the other person. Try not to respond straight away to what your partner says, listen instead to how he/she sees and experiences your relationship. Read your answers out loud to each other, taking turns to go first.

"I found it hard to answer all the questions before the second therapy session. Luckily my wife did too. We sat together complaining about our "homework". During the couple therapy sessions, some difficult topics came up that we hadn't spoken about since our children were born. For example, Kathy admitted how lonely she had felt since her miscarriage. I hadn't realised it then, because we already had two healthy children and I was convinced it would be fine the next time. That unprocessed grief of Kathy's and my lack of support for her clearly played a role in the difficult birth of our third child and the time just after it. My father was gravely ill then and I was preoccupied with renovating our house. In all the turmoil we started living parallel lives. Kathy, on the other hand, hadn't realised how deeply I had been affected by the death of my father. I didn't talk about it and she thought I didn't really need her support, because I didn't speak of my grief. Neither of us had been brought up to express our expectations and needs to each other, for fear of being disappointed or of sparking an argument. It's astonishing how naturally communication comes now since our trust in each other has been restored."
(Jeremy, 42 years old)

"The birth nearly took the lives of both Penny and Taylor (our baby boy). Before Taylor came along, we ran a successful advertising agency together. We had planned to take Taylor with us to the office, but in practice that happened very seldom. Penny gradually withdrew from the agency and her work was taken over by a number of interns. I could see how tired and tense she was and was walking on eggshells because I was afraid to add to her stress. In spite of this, we argued a couple of times a week, so hard that Penny once slammed a door so violently that the glass fell out of the frame. After fights like that we couldn't talk things through; after a few days of not talking at all, we carried on as if nothing had happened. Penny would go berserk if, for example, I stayed out after a football match to have a beer with my team. She thought it was very irresponsible of me now that I was a father, even though I went by bicycle and was still up early the following morning so that she could have a lie-in. I felt like I was quickly losing my freedom. When I took care of Taylor I could never do anything right by Penny. He was always dressed too warmly or not enough, or the clothes I had chosen didn't go together. It made me unsure of myself and I felt like I never had the chance to forge a bond with my son. I wanted to take him with me in the shower, but Penny was worried I would let him slip out of my hands. I wanted to go jogging in the woods with him in the buggy, but she thought that would put him at risk of Shaken Baby Syndrome.

Penny took a long time to recover physically from the birth, but her psychological recovery took much longer. I really thought I had lost her forever. When we saw a TV programme about PTSD following childbirth, we were both moved to tears. There was a name for what she was going through! The ensuing therapy made her feel much better. I began to see glimpses again of the women I fell in love with. Penny suggested we go to the coach together for a couple of sessions. I'm not very good at talking and feel very uncomfortable with all that 'irrational' stuff. But luckily I found the sessions to be very practical. In particular, the exercise where we had to describe an argument made many things clear to me. It made me understand that Penny was trying to make contact with me, even when she was annoyed with me. My reaction to her criticism was to run away, causing her, in turn to pursue me.

It turned out Penny was extra-sensitive to my drinking alcohol because her father drank too much in the past, causing tension between her parents. It was one of the reasons they eventually got divorced. I had had no idea that this was on her mind. She learned that a couple of beers on a Friday night were not the same as her father's former alcohol abuse. She understood that I needed those Friday evenings with my friends to relax and recharge. We went home with a diagram that set out exactly how Penny and I reacted to each other and how it could escalate. There was a clear pattern in our arguments. We became better at stopping the arguments from escalating and talked things through instead. Today we have a clear family set-up. Penny is involved in the advertising agency again. In the end, taking Taylor to the office with us didn't work out, so he goes to a crèche on the days that we're both at work." (Leon, 34 years old)

Exercise: Deconstructing an argument

Like Leon in the example above, you can also – separately – describe an argument you have had and see how you can ensure that a misunderstanding doesn't escalate, by taking a time-out before it's too late. You can do this by making a time-out gesture with your hands and then leaving the room.

- When you ....
....
....

(try to be as concrete as possible in describing/mentioning and without immediately blaming: snort, raise your eyebrow, say I should stop whining, don't want to have sex with me, are too busy at work, don't listen to me)

- then I react by/then I start ....
....
....

(complaining, freaking out, attacking, walking away, withdrawing, whining, becoming defensive)

- because I hope that you will then ....
....
....

(start listening to me, take me seriously, hold me, come after me, we won't fight anymore)

- When this happens I feel ....
....
....
(lonely, sad, afraid, ashamed, angry, furious, desperate, upset)

- And I see that you ....
....
....
(withdraw, walk away, counter-attack, disappear behind your computer, go out drinking with your friends, go jogging, put the television on, threaten to leave or divorce me, shut yourself off from me, shut down, pretend you don't care, act distant, avoid me, ignore me/refuse to talk to me.)

- The conclusion I draw about our relationship is ....
....
....
(I'm the only one working on it, it's over, you don't love me anymore, I can't count on you, I can't trust you, you don't listen to me, I feel shut out, I don't mean anything to you anymore, I'm not important to you, it would be better if we break up, you must have someone else).

"Men" versus "women"

Without wanting to run the risk of stereotyping, I have noticed during coaching sessions that women and men tend to react differently to problems in a relationship. I see that men, when faced with relationship problems, will more often:

- **feel they are inadequate** because they cannot resolve the relationship or communication problems;
- **become paralysed by all the emotions** and find this so disturbing that they prefer to bury their emotions and deny that there is a problem. Men feel "all sorts of things inside" but hide their feelings. Their partner often interprets this as a lack of feeling and becomes more irritated;
- **feel rejected.** Men like to have sexual intimacy to feel connected with their partner. Most women, on the other hand, want to first feel connected to their partner before they feel the desire for sex.

Men often react to problems or a crisis in their relationship by withdrawing from the relationship. They feel defeated or sad and grieve in silence for their relationship *("I can't do anything right at home anyway, I may as well walk away and bury myself in my work/hobby. At least there I matter/am appreciated.")*.
In this case it can help to focus on the bond you have with your child. It comes naturally to you to play with your baby, give her attention, touch, cuddle, comfort and care for her. You can apply this natural way of acting with your child(ren) to the way you behave with your partner.

As far as the typical woman is concerned (and, of course, there are exceptions), I've noticed in my practice that women tend to be more affected by:

- **loneliness and abandonment.** Their husband's life and work seems to continue as usual, while their own life is very different. Women often start working part-time, meaning that they take on a larger share of the childcare and household tasks;

- **feeling alone and loss of connection.** Women have a feeling they can't reach their partners and feel shut out, as if they are living with a roommate rather than a lover. They feel the need for "a good chat" and try to get their partner's attention by arguing;
- **lack of understanding.** They ask their partner to listen and respond on an emotional level and instead receive a concrete solution or rational piece of advice. The man feels that he has provided an answer, the women feels she hasn't had an answer. Both partners are correct, but on different levels, and both are frustrated.

If women don't get what they need from their male partners, they tend to share their feelings and sadness with other women. They feel connected to their women friends, and thus have less of a need to be connected with their partner.

Women's health seems to be closely linked to the emotional distance they have with their partner, while men's health is influenced by conflict and rejection. This often creates a vicious circle: decreasing feelings of affection leads to decreased intimacy (less or no sex), which leads to conflict, and in turn, a fear of abandonment. Because of this you are less willing to be vulnerable with your partner, you share less and this leads to a decrease in affection.

Sue Johnson asserts: *"When partners tell me that they cannot be considerate of and watch out for each other with everyday acts of caring, I worry. When they tell me that they are not making love, I am concerned. But when they tell me that they do not touch, I know they are really in trouble."* Hopefully, a couple can reverse this tide by speaking to a neutral third party, a therapist.

Recognising the raw spots or scars from your past

"We had no idea there was such a thing as 'raw spots or scars' left over from our youth and upbringing, let alone that they played a role in our current relationship problems. After our daughter was born, my very independent wife became possessive and insecure. She was afraid I would fall in love with another woman because she had not lost her pregnancy pounds and had moved her career down a slot. Because of the pregnancy pounds she didn't want to make love either and that made her terribly afraid I was going to move on to someone else. I felt like I was constantly giving her compliments, but my compliments seemed to disappear into a bottomless pit.

During the therapy session we realised that, as a child, Eva had never been complimented by her father. If she came home with good grades, she was told they should have been better; nothing was ever good enough. Crucially, when Eva was 17, her father ran off with his secretary and because of all the ensuing tension at home Eva failed her final exams. Her father saw this as a great shame. Eva then worked extra hard to gain recognition from her father. Since the birth she started working less and felt her father's disappointment and disapproval. I hadn't noticed this at all. On my side, I was used to settling my own issues, my way – that's how it had been in the large family I had grown up in. We never talked about feelings in our house. Since the birth Eva often wanted to talk about her feelings and about our relationship issues. I tried to escape. Eva became jealous and insecure. In the therapy sessions we learned that Eva was afraid of being abandoned just as she had been by her father. On one hand, I felt neglected because Eva was so preoccupied with her own problems and her recovery and, on the other hand, I couldn't stand her clinginess and jealousy. The more she followed me around and wanted to talk, the more I tried to escape from the house. The more I tried to make love to her to show her I was still attracted to her, the more she went to bed early to escape me and the intimacy. Once we were aware of this pattern, we were able to break it." (Bruno, 37 years old)

In the example above, Bruno talks about recognising raw spots or scars from your youth. You know it's a raw spot by the startlingly strong reaction from your partner to a seemingly (to you) small event. *"What's happened to you, suddenly? It wasn't that bad, was it?"* But it was that bad, because it touched on an old sore spot, an attachment need or an attachment fear: the attachment system was acutely activated. A look, a raised eyebrow, a remark, the tone in which something is said or a minor slur can be enough. Your body reacts immediately and powerfully, as a thunderbolt forces the limbic system over into survival mode, as if you're in a life-threatening situation. This is why for you there is suddenly a sense of alienation instead of connection between you.

You have already escaped or launched into an attack before you realise what is happening. Still, to discover and consciously feel raw spots and the accompanying fear is surprisingly "easier" than people think. You can help each other to identify them, so that they cease to play a role in your relationship or in an argument.

These are some questions you can ask yourself or your partner after an argument:
- What happened just before you got angry?
- What was the provocation?
- How did you feel? (afraid, angry, sad, distressed)
- What happened to your body? (blushing, trembling, heart palpitations, a headache, pain in your stomach)
- What went through your mind? (my partner doesn't understand me, finds me stupid, doesn't help or support me, I'm alone)
- What conclusion about yourself, your partner or your relationship did you draw at that moment? (I'm a loser, you're a..., here we go again, this will never get better, we should just break up)
- What did you need at that moment? What kind of (re)action did you long for? (comfort, understanding, a listening ear, a cup of tea, a massage, a time-out)

- With hindsight do you think this event/situation constitutes a raw spot from your childhood? Say what the situation makes you think about/reminds you of.
- What could your partner have done differently?

Obviously you can only ask your partner these questions once he or she has cooled down and is calm enough to listen with openness, empathy and curiosity. This is similar to the way you listen with interest on a first date to the story of somebody whom you would like to get to know better.

I would like to end this chapter with five golden tips to reinforce or improve the bond you have with your partner.

1. **Spend some time together as partners, not just parents.** Do things together, the more exciting, the better! If you experience something exciting together you both produce testosterone. This gives you butterflies and increases your libido (sex drive). So go bungee-jumping together, or parachuting, skydiving, deep-sea diving, kart racing, sailing or mountain biking.

2. **Celebrate your love.** Surprise each other with small thoughts: text messages, letters, a postcard or gift now and then, concert tickets or dinner at a restaurant. Take turns to arrange for a babysitter and think up an activity: from a walk on the beach to a movie, from going to see a play to a night in a hotel. The more you pay into your relationship "bank account", the higher the balance and the more you can deal with before you're "in the red".

3. **Listen to each other and make sure you are there for each other.** Even if you've heard all the stories about your partner's work and colleagues dozens of times, keep listening to his/her stories. Keep up to date with each other's doubts, difficulties at work, interesting projects and achievements, just as you do with your friends.

4. **Create special love rituals.** Mark important dates such as your wedding anniversary or Valentine's Day. Cherish the small things, such as a hug when you leave the house or

come home; Sunday breakfast as a family or bringing your partner a cup of coffee in bed when it's his/her turn to sleep late at the weekend.

5. **Give each other compliments, appreciation and recognition.** The power of this triple-treatment is all too often underestimated. Too many couples take each other for granted and forget to express their appreciation of each other or to give compliments regularly. They don't recognise how much their spouse does or how well they care for the children or for invalid parents. The greater the annoyance and irritations, the more compliments you need to restore the balance. Sincere compliments are the oil that keeps your relationship running smoothly. The more you give each other compliments (just like the small exchanges described in point 2 above), the higher you make the "bank balance" on your relationship account.

Peter's

STORY

I couldn't wait for our baby to be born. The pregnancy went well, we were really "pregnant together" and we followed antenatal classes together. Ingrid's contractions began a couple of days after the due date. The first stage of labour went well and the midwife complimented us on how well we were working together. Ingrid got in the bath and I sat next to her to time the contractions. When necessary I breathed together with her through the contractions or massaged her back. By the time the midwife returned, Ingrid was six centimetres dilated. Two hours later she was allowed to push. It took a long time, but finally, after an hour or so, the baby's head was born. I had expected the baby's body to come straight out after that – that's how it was in the films I'd seen – but nothing happened. Ingrid was completely unaware of it, but I saw the midwife exchange a look with the nurse and I knew: this was not right. Then I saw the baby's head start to turn blue. My heart was beating in my throat. The midwife called to the nurse to phone for an ambulance. I shouted: *"I'll do it!"* because I wanted to be useful. It felt like hours before I was connected with the emergency services. I couldn't get my words out and the nurse took over the phone. Afterwards, the midwife told me she had given me a direct line to call but in the panic I hadn't heard her. I felt like such a loser: I had left my wife's side and hadn't even been able to call an ambulance.

The baby was born quite soon after that. The midwife gave him oxygen and he was soon a healthy pink colour. I heard the ambulance sirens in the street. The paramedics came upstairs, saw that the situation was under control and left again.
A couple of hours later, Ingrid and Karl – our baby boy –

were both asleep. I, however, was wide awake. That night I hardly closed my eyes. Images of the birth haunted me, especially Karl's blue face between my wife's legs. I broke out in a cold sweat whenever I thought about it.

Over the next few days I tried to talk to Ingrid about the birth. She had experienced it very differently. When I asked her why she thought the midwife had called for an ambulance, she replied: *"Oh, just as a caution."* I didn't want to upset her with my story – I had the feeling anyway that I had been completely useless from the moment the panic set in. In the week after the birth I hardly slept. Nobody asked how the birth had gone for me: they only asked Ingrid, while I was there. Her account was very positive. She was very proud to have been able to deliver Karl at home. How could I then force my horror story into the picture? Her experience was much more important than mine, wasn't it? So I didn't say anything... I began to dread night-time, but I couldn't say anything about that either. A week after the birth I was back at work, but I could barely concentrate.

Ingrid went alone to the postnatal meeting with the midwife. She went alone to the medical check-ups for the baby. I needed all my energy to stay on my feet and to pretend at work and at home that everything was alright. After a couple of months, Ingrid tried to get close again but I was unable to be intimate with her. I kept seeing Karl's blue head between her legs. I hated myself for this and couldn't tell her why I wasn't getting aroused. I pretended I was tired from work and from the broken nights we had because of the baby. Ingrid said she didn't mind but I felt like an impotent old man. You always hear about women not wanting to have sex after giving birth, but with us it was the other way around. Six months later there was organisational restructuring at my work. That was the last straw for me. I broke down and called in sick. My doctor gave me sleeping pills for a week because I hadn't slept properly for six months, and advised me to speak to a therapist. When she asked how the birth had gone, I gave her Ingrid's and the midwife's version. Then she asked: *"And how was it for you? What was your experience?"* Before I knew what was happening, I was weeping like a small child, with big noisy sobs – it was mortifying. After that I felt a huge weight lift off me.

She suggested I try out EMDR (see Chapter 7). During the EMDR session the image of Karl's dangling blue head came back to me. The thought I associated with it was "I'm failing" and I felt afraid, powerless and sad. My shoulders were cramped during the session and I thought my head would explode from the tension. But quite soon after that the tension dropped and the image faded, as if I were looking at it through a kind of see-through mirror on the wall. At the end of it, even my wristwatch was broken on the inside. The session ended with a relaxation exercise and I felt a difference in my neck and shoulders straight away. After six months, I suddenly had a neck again, my head wasn't stuck straight on to my torso anymore.

In another coaching session I "redid" the birth, as it were. That might sound vague or wishy-washy, but it was great. I pictured myself sitting behind Ingrid, just as I had been before it all went wrong. And just like in a film, Karl slipped easily out of her. The midwife gave Karl to Ingrid, who held him against her chest, while I held my wife and my child tightly. How good that felt! I cried again but this time they were happy tears. In my version of the birth, I got to hold Karl after that while Ingrid was stitched up. I could almost feel him against my skin while I was sitting in the coach's office. She advised me to have a bath with Karl at some point and to tell him this version of the birth story. I'm not really a bath person, but I did take him with me in the shower. That was the last time I cried. He watched me, incredibly naturally, as if he knew exactly what I was going through. A couple of weeks later I was back at work. I kept my job in spite of the restructuring and my temporary breakdown. Nowadays, my sleep has become lighter than before the birth, but other fathers seem to have that effect too. Our sex life has slowly recovered as well – we're now trying for a second baby.

I'm telling you my story, because I hope it will strike a chord with you, so you might be able to tell someone your story too: even if your story is different from your wife's story, and even if nobody asks for your version.

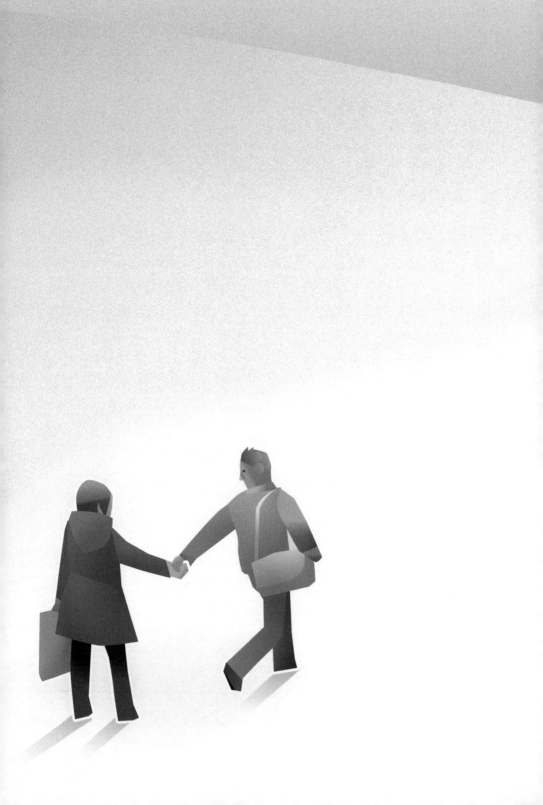

CHAPTER 6

When your child passes away during your pregnancy or around the time of the birth

Around 1% of babies die during pregnancy or around the time of birth. The death of a baby around the time of birth cannot be compared to the other distressing births described in this book. That's why I've included this chapter for parents who, in addition to having to process a traumatic birth, are dealing with their grieving process and bearing the unbearable: the loss of a much-desired child. If the baby dies during pregnancy, your labour will start spontaneously or will be induced after a few days. Because a C-section is an operation that carries a number of risks, including for subsequent pregnancies, babies who die in the womb are usually born vaginally. In consultation with the mother, this can happen with or without an epidural. In English, the term stillbirth is used – unfortunately an apt description. When I worked as a midwife, I oversaw a number of births of deceased babies.

There is often a deafening stillness during and after such a birth. In contrast, when a baby dies unexpectedly during labour, there is panic, fear and a cacophony of sounds and impressions. It's hard to imagine that so much can happen in a short space of time and how the lives of the parents-to-be are so quickly turned upside-down..

"I was at work when I suddenly started to lose blood. Two weeks earlier I had had an amniocentesis because the combined test revealed a high risk of Down's syndrome. I knew straight away that something wasn't right. My colleague drove me to the hospital where they confirmed that my baby had indeed died. I don't remember exactly what the doctors told me, other than that I should call my husband and give him the impossible news. A few days later they induced my labour. The birth was hell. I didn't want to give birth – and certainly not to a dead baby. And the baby apparently didn't want to be born either: I laboured for two days until Sarah finally arrived. I caught a fever and felt as sick as a dog. All the time I was lying in the maternity ward, I could hear other women and their babies. It was so incredibly painful. In the last phase of the birth there were five people around my bed, but almost none of them did or said anything. There was no encouragement, and of course there was no need to listen for a heartbeat. I didn't speak either – for almost two days. There was nothing to say.

When Sarah was born they placed her on my stomach. I couldn't bear the thought of that beforehand, but now I'm happy that they did it. She was perfect – her body was fully formed. Because I couldn't deliver the placenta I had to have an operation anyway. When I was in the operating room I began to panic and everything became too much. Since I was in a panic when I went under, I still felt panicked when I came out of the general anaesthetic. The amniocentesis showed that Sarah had been healthy after all. I felt so terribly guilty that I had agreed to the amniocentesis, even though all the doctors told me her death was unrelated to it. When my coach asked if the guilt was halting my ability to process the experience, I felt a shock wave through my body. I had indeed been torturing myself every day with 'why?' and 'if only I had... if only I hadn't...' The first therapy session focused therefore on taking the blame off myself. I had listened to the doctors' advice and followed it precisely. There was no need to blame myself.

After that, we dealt with the feelings of panic. When we talked about the episode in the operating room, I almost passed out and started hyperventilating. After two days of thinking only of delivering the baby, I was finally able to see and hold Sarah. I didn't want to let her go. I didn't want the general anaesthetic. I fought against myself and my sense of panic grew. With hindsight, I think they should have calmed and reassured me before they put me under. I also 'lost' whole sections of the birth. My partner, Tom, was not allowed in the operating room. When I came round I was screaming and shaking. I was only allowed to go to Tom once I had calmed down. Afterwards I thought it would have been nice if Tom had been allowed to be with me in the recovery room. I had felt so alone. My teeth were chattering so hard I couldn't drink out of a glass and needed a straw. When I was taken back to the room, my parents were there, as well as my sister, Tom's parents, his brother and sister-in-law. It was much too much for me. I wanted everyone to just go away. I wanted to be alone with Sarah and Tom. At the same time I was glad our families were there and had a chance to see Sarah. It was all so confusing. It felt good to discuss all the pieces of the 'Sarah puzzle' with my coach and to notice that I felt a little lighter after each session. Being in mourning is terrible. People think you're still pregnant; at work they didn't understand that I was taking 'birth leave'. The work doctor called it 'sick leave' but I stubbornly referred to it as birth leave because that was how it felt to me. The worst part was when I saw people I knew in the supermarket or on the street and they swiftly turned their heads or crossed the road, pretending they hadn't seen me. They did anything to avoid having to talk to me. I would have preferred for them to say that they didn't know what to say – anything would have been better than being avoided. Losing your child is awful; the unhelpful behaviour of the people around you makes it extra painful.

I can't imagine having got through that period without professional help – it was just too big, too painful, too all-encompassing. I needed someone to keep telling me that what I was going though was normal, that my reaction was understandable, that somehow it was all going to be alright. I watched as one friend after another become pregnant, and each time it stung right through to my heart. I was happy for them, but each time it threw back in my face the fact that I didn't have Sarah. I thought I would never recover from it, but in the end I made my way out. I gave Sarah a place in my heart and in my life. She isn't here but I 'speak' to her regularly. She now has a little brother, Job. When I heard him cry for the first time – just the fact that he made a sound when he was born – it was the most beautiful music I'd ever heard." (Stella, 27 years old)

> The loss of a child is a primeval loss that can't be compared to any other kind of loss. Where are you supposed to find the strength to bear the unbearable? You hadn't even – or hardly even – had the chance to meet your baby when you were forced

to say goodbye. During the pregnancy you probably already forged an attachment to your child; you already loved your baby. When you lost him, you also lost your vision of the future. You had already pictured yourself pushing a pram or sitting under a Christmas tree together. Your heart is overflowing with love, but your womb is empty, the pram is empty and so are your arms... There is a child who will forever be in your heart, whom you will love forever but whom you won't be caring for every day. The writer PF Thomése, who lost his small daughter, describes this very poignantly in his book *Shadow Child:*
"A woman who lives longer than her husband is called a widow, a man without his wife a widower. A child without parents is an orphan. But what do you call the father and mother of a child who has died?"

Swinging back and forth between grief and trust

The Dual Process Model of Coping with Bereavement from psychologists Stroebe and Schut gives insight into the life of a person in mourning. In this model, there are two circles. The first circle gives attention to dealing with the loss. This includes grieving but also being sad, ruminating and having feelings of disbelief, denial, avoidance and anger. The other circle focuses on healing and describes the search for a new balance in your life, starting new relationships and dealing with stress stemming from a changed life vision. You have become parents but don't have a baby to look after. Instead of the scientific model, I've decided to fill the two circles in this book with words that I've heard my clients use. When you lose your child, you swing back and forth between sorrow and anxiety on one hand (the left circle) and hope and trust on the other hand (the right circle).

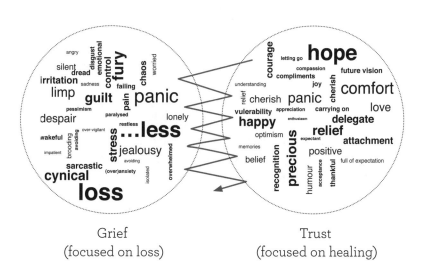

Grief
(focused on loss)

Trust
(focused on healing)

Parents often say they feel guilty when they laugh, go out for dinner, exercise, go on holiday again, and take their minds off their deceased baby for a while. With the help of the two circles in the diagram, I explain to them that this is completely normal. As a grieving parent you cannot grieve continuously.
The pain and sadness are too intense for that to be possible. Your body and mind regularly need a time-out to recharge. When confronted with your sorrow, it's normal to look for distraction to escape the distress for a while. Sometimes you do this consciously and feel clearly "I don't want to be sad right now", sometimes you are unaware that it's happening. Pushing away negative emotions takes a lot of energy and eventually you pay the price with your health. It can have all kinds of physical and psychological repercussions.

Understandably, in the first stage of the grieving process, most people focus on their loss (in the left circle) and their emotions are very raw. With time, the focus gradually shifts to recovery (the right circle) and finding a new balance in life. Sometimes it helps to "park" your sorrow for a while by consciously distracting yourself from it. A couple of days off can help you avoid letting your bereavement wear you out completely. You aren't running away from your sorrow by doing this, you are taking a moment to recharge, so that you can face it again later when you have more energy. Don't worry about what outsiders might think if you do something fun or if you smile, if it helps you. If you notice that you (or your partner) are entirely focused on your loss, or, on the contrary, are trying to move on with your life, you may need some extra support with your grieving process. For example, you can try to seek contact with other parents who have also lost their child. People who have been through a similar experience understand better what you are going through and listen differently to your story.

Contact with fellow sufferers can take place in physical gatherings as well as through online support groups. One advantage of online groups is that they are also available at night. Frequently, you won't be the only parent-of-a-deceased-child who is online when they are unable to sleep.

If you prefer to have extra support from a healthcare professional, you can contact a coach or therapist specialising in bereavement. Ask your doctor or midwife to refer you to someone who has experience with guiding parents who have lost a child, or ask other parents to recommend someone they had a good rapport with.

"It felt so good to realise that I was in the positive circle more and more often and for longer. When I reread my gratefulness diary, I noticed I was making small steps. I had more understanding for myself when I found myself sinking back into the sorrow-and-fear circle. I was getting better at embracing my sorrow. The more I embraced it, the sooner the crying fits would pass. The other thing I learned was to call upon my sorrow. Sometimes I felt it coming while I was at the office. I pushed it away because I didn't want to cry at work. At the end of the day I went home with a terrible headache from holding back my tears. And when I was finally allowed to cry, the tears didn't come. I learned how to 'summon' the sorrow by sitting in my baby's room and holding a soft toy (the same as the one we put into his coffin), or by listening to the music we played at his funeral. I also received a lot of support from an online group we found through the hospital. This played a big part at night, at weekends and on holidays such as Christmas when everyone else was celebrating with their families. There is no group so united as one that brings together people who share such a dreadful experience. Nonetheless, even that group was sometimes too much for me: such terrible stories, especially from people who had been in the group for years and still spoke as if they had only just lost their child. It really seemed to me like I needed somebody else at every stage of recovery.

I processed the birth so that I would be able to separate it in my mind from my son, Tim, himself. Tim died from a heart defect that had nothing to do with the birth, but I had bundled the two together in my mind because, before he was born he was 'normal', with a good strong heartbeat, according to the midwife. I also learned to feel my feelings and to talk about them. I had always thought I could talk easily but surprised myself when it came to learning to express my sadness and fear. The more I spoke to others about Tim, the easier it became to cry about it. A new colleague who was childless by choice once made an unintentionally painful remark: *'Have you also chosen not to have children because of your career?'* I burst into tears to the amazement of my colleagues. They said they had no idea I was *'still in that place'* because I *'never talked about it'*. Interesting… I blamed my colleagues for not asking about Tim and they didn't want to mention him for fear of upsetting me. Now I'm able to just say: *'Oh, I wish I could do that with Tim'*, and even if it makes me cry, nobody minds. A colleague of mine said recently that, thanks to me and Tim, he was able to respond very differently to his sister-in-law when she had a miscarriage. I find it special that other people can learn something because I shared my story." (Eve, 32 years old)

Different ways of grieving

During my coaching sessions, I give attention not only to the way the mother is processing her loss, but also how her partner, parents, family and friends are coping with it. Everyone has their own way of dealing with sorrow and loss. It's important to understand that your loved ones might have a different way of processing such an event. If you expect others to do things exactly as you do, you risk being extremely disappointed. Try to put yourself in the other person's shoes, see if you understand what they're trying to tell you and make it clear to them also how you feel and what you need. Looking at how people deal with great loss, we can roughly distinguish two ways.

The first group of people has the need to share and express their feelings. They spend more time in the left circle and mainly display emotions such as sadness, guilt, anger and fear. They need understanding, sympathy and moral support from the people around them. This is called an "emotion-focused coping style". Emotion-focused coping is effective in situations that don't change, such as the death of a baby. While the first group focuses on being sad, the second group mostly has the need to do something. After the loss of a child, they prefer to concentrate on healing (the right circle) rather than loss (the left circle). They don't feel like talking about painful subjects such as the loss of their baby, because *"it's bad enough as it is"*, and *"talking about it doesn't solve the problem"*. They want to work actively to address the problem. This is called a "problem-focused coping style". It's extremely effective in situations that can be influenced or resolved, but unfortunately the death of a baby doesn't fall into that category. If you and your partner have different ways of coping there can be communication problems. I help clients to concentrate on what they have in common: both parents are grieving and feeling intense sorrow. Understanding for each other's way of grieving prevents partners from losing each other in a negative bereavement spiral, which can come about when one of the partners only sees their own grieving process and therefore cannot have understanding for their partner's "different" way of grieving.

"As if it weren't bad enough that we had lost our child... Nearly a year after our first baby Fiona died, my husband Ed and I were on the verge of losing each other. We didn't understand each other anymore; we were handling our bereavement in completely different ways and couldn't reach each other. Because of all the arguing we didn't even make love anymore, even though we both wanted a second child so badly. I processed the first birth experience, which made a huge impression on me. I wanted to share my experience with Ed but he wasn't interested. While I slowly started to feel better, he was getting worse. He started hyperventilating and ended up home on sick leave.

The coach asked if Ed would be willing to go and tell his story. I would never have expected it, but he went. When he came home from the coaching session his eyes were completely swollen and he went straight to bed. I had to bite my tongue to stop myself from asking about it. I heard from Ed's parents, brother and best friend how he had experienced Fiona's birth: how dreadful it was for him to watch as they tried to resuscitate her, how it took almost a year to get that image out of his head and for the nightmares to cease.

In the hope of avoiding the terrifying nightmares, he drank too much in the evening and stayed up half the night playing games on his laptop. I literally had no idea what he had been going through. I often criticised him for his drinking and that made him withdraw even more behind his laptop. He didn't want to talk to me, but luckily we did manage to talk when we were with the coach. I was shocked during a coaching session when he tearfully admitted that he was afraid of starting another pregnancy because he couldn't face the chance of losing another child. He told me he sometimes started an argument purposely so that I wouldn't want to have sex with him and thus risk another pregnancy.

I took him in my arms and felt closely connected to him. We shared our sadness about Fiona's death, even though our way of expressing that sadness was so different. We learned to really talk to each other, including about painful emotions and about what we needed from each other. They were very different conversations from the kind we had had before Fiona. We learned that it's completely normal to sway back and forth between fear and longing. We waited until the longing was greater than the fear – for both of us – before we tried for a new baby. We are now more than four years on and have a little boy, Theo, and a baby girl, Manu. Fiona will always be our eldest child – she made us parents." (Ed, 40 years old and Karin, 38 years old)

The grieving process: your grief, your way

You mourn someone whom you loved or with whom you had a special bond. It isn't the length but the depth of your love that counts here. It's almost impossible to feel no pain at all when you lose someone whom you loved very much. I see grieving and love as two sides of the same coin.

Grieving is not a disease but you can literally become "sick" with grief. People who have suffered intense loss almost always score as depressed on a depression screening test. It's sometimes difficult for bystanders and even healthcare providers to tell the difference between grief and depression.

If a woman who has lost her baby feels down, listless and sorrowful, she will be diagnosed – sometimes incorrectly – with postpartum (postnatal) depression.

Your mourning isn't "over" after a year. Most people say they didn't get over the loss of their child but that they managed, with the help of their family, friends and sometimes external support, to get through the horrific period. Grief is like a shadow: it's always there, sometimes bigger, sometimes invisible. You might sometimes be in darkness, sometimes hardly aware of the shadow and then suddenly overwhelmed by it.

Grief is not usually characterised by a continuous feeling of depression but more by sudden, intense throbs of sorrow. You can be suddenly and unexpectedly hurled back to the left circle when you were in the right one. With time, the frequency of the painful onslaughts might lessen while the intensity will remain the same.

There are no protocols for dealing with bereavement. Other people can't tell you how you "must" process your loss or how you "must" feel. It's your bereavement, your sorrow, your grieving process. You can only do it your way. Take as much time as you need, let others know what your needs are, do whatever feels good for you and do it your way. Grieving has two parts: acknowledging your feelings and working towards healing. It helps to regularly allow yourself some distraction from your sadness. Surround yourself with people who support you and bring you what you need. Friends and family can also sometimes give you a gentle and loving push in the right direction.

Many people seem to know what's best for you, while you yourself don't know what is good and what isn't. You don't have to follow well-intentioned advice from others unless it feels right for you. If somebody gives you unwanted advice, thank them for their advice or opinion and just let the "good advice" slide off you as best you can. You can ask others to listen to you and tell them how you feel and how you're dealing with your loss. You often get more recognition by allowing yourself to be vulnerable with people who are important to you and by telling them what you're going through. This helps you and makes it easier for others to stay involved in your grieving process. Keep listening to yourself, follow your intuition and do what feels good at that precise moment, because every day is different. In one day you might feel good at one point, and an hour later have the feeling that nothing will be right again. This is completely normal. You can't avoid that you sometimes feel overtaken by grief and the pain of your loss. Unfortunately, the people around you and society often react differently towards you when you've lost a child. There is a big difference between the life of parents with children and that of parents who have lost their baby and you will sometimes mistakenly be put in the category of childless couples.

The power of mourning rituals

In the old days there was a series of mourning rituals, such as mourning clothes that were worn for one year, a wake and religious remembrance services, to display your loss to the outside world. Nowadays mourning has become invisible. Nobody sees that you are suffering inside and falling apart from sorrow. If you don't cry, it seems as if your sorrow doesn't exist. For outsiders it's sometimes easier to pretend they don't see your grief, because if they see it, they feel they need to do something about it... and most people have no idea how to act with parents who have lost a child. Your world has come to a stop, while the rest of the world seems to just keep on going, unaffected. You can choose to come up with your own rituals, for example, by choosing a symbol that represents your loss or by holding a parting or remembrance gathering for your baby. I know parents who organise such a gathering every year, in order to keep the memory of their baby "alive". Mourning rituals can help you with what the Germans appropriately call "mourning work" *(Trauerarbeit)*. To mourn is hard work. It explains why you might be so tired during the grieving process, even though you have the impression you're not doing anything. Integrating grief into your life takes a lot of energy and time. It's normal to make mistakes occasionally. It's normal that the tapestry of your life will have some holes after you have lost a child.

Once again: take as much time as you need! Do it your way: that's the only way. By living through the pain and sorrow you will be able to carry on with your life. Certain moments can be extra tough. For example, feast days might well feel like days of mourning – on those days, feelings of sorrow and loss of a much-desired baby are greatest. Don't make any advance plans for those days. See how you feel and what you need on the day itself, who you would like to be with, or even, if you would like to be alone. An increasing number of hospitals organise annual memorial get-togethers where all the babies who died that year in that hospital are remembered by name. The second Sunday in December is Worldwide Candle Lighting Day. At 7pm, people all over the world light a candle to remember the children they have lost.

"Every year my friends come together on Simon's birth- and death day. We've been doing it for three years now. I don't need to remind my friends, they are there, just as they have always been there since Simon's birth and death. When I hear about other parents in my situation, I realise how lucky we are to have the friends we do. We didn't lose any of them when Simon died. Every year on the anniversary of his birth and death, we meet at 4pm by his grave, we hug each other and then we go out for a drink together."
(Zoe, 28 years old)

Disbelief and denial are part of the process

It often takes some time before the loss completely hits you. You "know" that it happened but it seems so unreal, like a bad dream. It can't be true. Why is this happening to us? It's important to face the situation, to see your baby, so that you can convince yourself that it isn't a dream. It's a good idea to hold your baby and to give him/her a name. It might also help for your loved ones to meet your child. The more people there are who know your baby, the easier it will be for you to talk about him/her. It's normal to find it hard to believe and sometimes even to deny what happened to you. It's normal to feel desperate, powerless and hopeless; it's also normal to feel nothing at all. If your child suffered before his death you might also feel relieved that the suffering is over. But you can also feel guilty about it. Find people with whom you can share these emotions. Don't be frightened by the intensity of your emotions. All feelings want is to be felt. Very often, people in mourning try to bury their pain or sorrow by using alcohol, drugs, medication, overworking, sports or binge-eating. In the short term these can be effective solutions to numb the pain, but in the long run they will work against you. You are adding to your problems instead of giving attention to the cause.

If emotions and feelings are "allowed" without anyone finding it strange or being judgemental about it (yourself included), they will become less powerful with time. Many parents describe it as an empty feeling inside, a silence around them, or that being surrounded by people makes them feel lonelier than ever.

"I couldn't believe it when, a few days after the birth of our son, Storm, who died inside me at 23 weeks of pregnancy, my mother-in-law tearfully revealed that she had also lost a baby at almost six months of pregnancy. Even my husband hadn't known about it. How differently it had been for her nearly 40 years ago. She had given birth under a sheet and had never been offered the chance to see or hold her baby, let alone give it a name. When she held Storm in her arms in the hospital I saw her break down, but I didn't know that her sadness was twice as great. She was crying for Storm but also for her own baby. With help from my coach, my mother-in-law was able to symbolically say goodbye to her baby, because no child can be missed as one who is no longer there. She made a box and put into it a short poem, a stone shaped like a heart, and a soft toy. Then, she went up to the dunes, alone, where she buried the box as a symbol. She wanted to do it alone because she had given birth alone and had carried her grief alone all those years. I'm so glad I was able to hold Storm, that we could take his footprints and that we were allowed to bury him ourselves (also in the dunes)." (Michelle, 35 years old)

From my clients I often hear that the worst moment in the day is when they wake up in the morning because then they still think that everything is "normal". Just after that, the reality of their loss stabs through them and they are overtaken by a flood of grief. It's normal for your loss to flow over you in waves and that these waves are summoned by smells, sounds or images that remind you of your pregnancy, delivery or baby. The smallest experiences or (unthought-through) remarks from others can suddenly produce deep feelings of sorrow. When you feel overwhelmed or overtaken by grief, it can help you to express your feelings no matter where or with whom you are at that moment. Usually people have no idea what is happening to you in that moment. If someone says something that is very painful for you, you can just say *"Ouch!"* out loud. You would also say that if you bump your knee in a painful way or if someone collides hard into you. So if someone smashes into your heart with their words, you can just as well say *"Ouch"*. Everybody would understand. If you express your pain using the Four-part Nonviolent Communication method given in Chapter 5, people around you can be aware of it:

I hear/see that you are saying ....
(= **put into words** what you see/hear)
How do you mean that? What do you want to say?
(= ask for what they **mean**)

That gives me a feeling of ....
and I find it unpleasant/painful/that hurts me.
(= **realise** and say what it does to you)
I need you to/I would prefer you to say/do ....
(= what you **need**)

Stay as close as possible to your own feeling and be as clear
as possible about what you need. The clearer your request (for
help), the easier it will be for others to respond concretely and
to fulfil that specific need.

"Five days after she was born, our daughter Danielle died from a very
rare inherited metabolic disorder. My husband and I are both healthy,
but tests following Danielle's death showed that we are both carriers
of the gene that causes the metabolic disorder that killed her. Because
of this there is a 25% chance that our next child will also have the
disorder and will also die a few days after birth.

For me the worst thing was that everybody told me I was coping
well and that I was so strong. They meant it well but it made it
much harder to admit that I was actually not strong at all and that I
was sometimes not coping at all. Together with the coach I looked
through the happy photos from just after the birth. Ruud and I still
thought then that our baby was healthy. We looked so happy on those
few photos. After that we looked at the photos that a professional
photographer took of us and Danielle after she passed away.
Danielle died in our arms – which is the most unimaginable thing
to go through. We told her: *'You came to us out of love and we're now
letting you go again out of love.'* We took her home with us and our
close family members came to see her. We made a photo report: five
valuable photos and a DVD with 120 photos, what a precious memory
of our daughter and what a special 'proof' of ourselves as parents
with Danielle in our arms. We found a specially made baby book with
beautiful illustrations and fitting quotations and poems, because a
standard baby book isn't appropriate when your child has passed away.

Several of my friends, my sister and three sisters-in-law had been
pregnant at the same time as me, so there were babies being born one
after the other all around us. That was difficult. I began to withdraw

more and more and stayed away from parties and birthdays, because I wasn't able to be strong anymore. I went quiet when people made painful comments, while I'm usually very chatty. Sorting out the administration around the baby and having to cancel my maternity leave were additional torments. People not wanting or daring to talk about Danielle was (and still is) very painful. I learned that there would be days when I was 'strong' and days when I was 'not strong', as well as days when I was strong and sad at the same time. I learned to ask for support and to receive it; before Danielle was born I was usually the one giving support to others. I learned to express what I was feeling, what I was thinking and what I needed from people around me when things were bleak. This turns out to be much harder when you're going through a rough time than in more cheerful times. It was wonderful that my husband, Ruud, was also involved in the healing process. Luckily, we made it through together, each in our own way. Danielle's arrival and departure taught us to communicate differently and to see other sides of each other. The fact that we endured and survived this together makes us feel that we can face anything together, for the rest of our lives.

We're now expecting our second baby, a little brother or sister for Danielle. We already know that this baby doesn't have the terrible metabolic disease that took Danielle. The pregnancy is certainly not a peaceful experience. I keep wavering between hope and dread. When I cry about Danielle I feel guilty towards the baby growing in me. During this pregnancy I have been getting psychological care as well as the usual medical care, and this has been very helpful. I've learned that I can tell the baby that my tears are for his/her older sister and that my sadness has nothing to do with him/her. Sorrow can exist alongside joy. Some days this works better than others. I can't wait to hold our healthy baby in my arms." (Nicole, 31, and Ruud, 33 years old)

Understanding what happened

Nicole and Ruud know what their baby daughter died from. This can be a source of worry but can also give you security. While Nicole and Ruud knew there was a high risk of it happening again, they also know their second child doesn't have the illness. Bereavement expert Manu Keirse says: *"We can't process loss. We process waste. With loss, you need to learn to live with it. You learn to incorporate it into your life."* In order to be able to incorporate your experience of loss in your life in the long term, it might help to understand what exactly happened and how it was possible.

You can start by collecting as much information as you can from the doctors or midwives. If this is still too hard for you, you can ask someone to help you do it or even to do it for you. It's possible to make an appointment, even months later, with the healthcare provider who was present at the birth of your child. When the worst of the pain has lessened it's often easier to place information. Wait until you're ready. If, at a later stage you have additional questions you can make a new appointment if necessary. When making the appointment, inform them that your child died at the time of birth, so that the doctor or midwife schedules extra time to talk to you. If you don't get clear answers to your questions, keep looking for an explanation that is satisfactory to you. Unfortunately, in some cases you will never get the answers you need. If no cause of death has been found, the risk of it happening again is usually also smaller. This can give you comfort and hope.

"We never found out the reason Jack died in my belly. That was extra hard for me, as a scientist who always wants to understand. If something wasn't clear to me in the past, I would buy books, read studies online or ask experts for an explanation, until I understood. Unfortunately, there was nothing to understand about Jack's death. He was perfect, everything in the right place. No explanation was revealed by the autopsy or the examination of the placenta. I had a healthy lifestyle, I didn't drink or smoke, my blood pressure was just right – and still he died. The doctor in the hospital called his death 'bad luck'. For a long time that stuck in my throat. The coaching journey was heavy and intense with many low points but also a high point. During the EMDR session I realised – once I had cleared away my sadness and fury – how much love I had felt for Jack just after he was born. Those eyelashes, those nails, that cleft chin (like mine), his father's nose, those ears, that hair… All that had disappeared under the blanket of horror during the birth and once I had got that blanket out of my system, only love was left.

When I think back to Jack's stillbirth now, it's the love that predominates. Jack taught me that life isn't fixable, that not everything is possible with hard work and determination. That not everything can be understood and how incredibly hard it is to accept that his death was unexplainable. But going around in circles and ruminating didn't help either – it wasn't going to bring him back.

I didn't dare get pregnant again until I had a satisfactory explanation for Jack's death. But during my coaching journey, I did get pregnant again. Physically, the pregnancy went well, but psychologically it was a very difficult time. I fought every day to remain positive, to believe in the power of my healthy body and in the life strength of this baby. Only when I held Emma in my arms did it all come out. We actually spent three days alone at home, just the three of us. Only the visiting nurse was in the background. For three days, we watched Emma with wonder, cried and told her about her older brother." (Kathleen, 35 years old)

Physical complaints

When you're in mourning you can get all kinds of physical symptoms. You can literally feel empty, or on the contrary, have so much pressure in your chest that you fear you might have a heart attack. You might suffer from insomnia, listlessness, lack of appetite or binge-eating. This can lead to digestive and stomach problems. Head, neck and back pain are also common. These complaints are often present in the first months following a heavy loss but can also only appear months later. To ease your physical and tension-related complaints, try massage, yoga, mindfulness or the tips given at the end of Chapter 3. If your physical complaints last much longer, you should consult a doctor. This doesn't apply to insomnia. If you really sleep much less than you're used to and this is negatively impacting your ability to function during the day, then it's advisable to contact your doctor after one week.

Anger

The pain of loss can also show itself through belligerence and aggressiveness. You might feel angry at everyone, yourself, your loved ones, God, the doctors or the hospital. It's important not to hold back these feelings but to let them out. Sometimes people around you might want to protect you (or themselves) from these violent emotions, but these feelings should also be allowed to exist. Thoughts such as "What have we done to deserve this?" or "Nobody understands what I'm going through" are normal. Express them, so that your loved ones know what's going on inside you. Often, your loved ones will be doing everything wrong and you'll take your frustrations out on them. You'll feel stifled when they're around too much and angry when they don't contact you or don't talk about your loss. This can lead to conflict situations: they want the best for you and you don't want to offend anyone. It might also happen that they avoid the topics of pregnancy, motherhood or babies in order to protect you. This might mean that you're the last to find out that a friend is pregnant. This doesn't help most women – on the contrary. Let your friends and family know where you stand and what your needs are, as well as how you would like to hear the "good news". This could be in an email, for example, so that you have time to process it and then, in your own time, when you're ready, call your friend to congratulate her. When you visit friends and their newborns, it's also good if there is room for the joy of the new parents as well as for your own sadness and regret. Explain that it helps if you can describe yourself how you're feeling rather than having others tell you how you should be feeling. You're not looking for pity, you're sad. Sometimes, a mother might give you her baby to hold, thinking it will comfort you, other times, everyone will get to hold the baby, except you. Both these situations can be painful and confrontational. Think in advance what you believe would be easiest for you on each specific day for each specific visit, and discuss this, where possible, before you go there.

Guilt

Guilt is useful to a certain extent. It helps to make your puzzle complete and encourages you to think about whether you could have done something to prevent your baby's death. If you're able to ask yourself this question and to answer it honestly, the feeling of guilt usually fades by itself.

If, in spite of this, you find that you're still bearing a lot of guilt and that you keep brooding "if only I had..." and "what if...", the questions below might help you.

- Is what you believe true (whatever you're feeling guilty about)?
- Is there information missing? And if so, who can tell you more about it?
- How do you feel (what happens to you) when you believe this thought?
- How would you feel without those thoughts/feelings?

Feelings of guilt can hold you prisoner and trap you in a cycle of rumination. Unfortunately, this doesn't solve anything (see Chapter 2). If your baby died during, or as a result of, the birth, your feeling of guilt is often mingled with the (unjustified) feeling of guilt of the doctor or midwife. All this guilt stands in the way of an objective view of the event and an objective discussion between parents and healthcare providers.

It can help to have an impartial third person in the room (see Chapter 1 on the importance of the postnatal discussion).

Faith

Your faith and world view can also change as a result of your loss. People who were brought up to be religious can derive solid support from their faith. However, it can also happen that their loss takes away their ability to believe in God or Allah. Atheists, on the other hand, might acquire a spiritual awareness, perhaps because they felt the presence or nearness of their baby after his/her passing. A change in life convictions can turn your life even more upside-down, because those around you can also think differently about it.

What helps and what doesn't help

Just as with other unpleasant events, it can help to write down your experience, as explained in Chapter 2. Make it clear to the people around you what you expect from them. Unfortunately, a lack of understanding from their loved ones often seems to be part of the "parcel" that grieving parents are given. Many clients express frustration that they can't bring themselves to "educate" their friends and family about what they should and shouldn't say... For most people there is no lack of willingness but rather a lack of knowledge and ability.

Listening

When somebody in your circle is going through a period of mourning, it's normal to not always know how to deal with it. Remember one thing: the greatest gift you can bring to a grieving person is to listen to their story. The Chinese symbol for listening is therefore so appropriate.

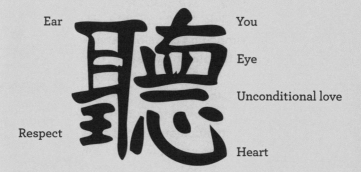

Ear

Respect

You

Eye

Unconditional love

Heart

It's made up of various symbols that separately mean eye, ear, you, respect, unconditional love and heart. Isn't that beautiful? If you have a friend who has lost a child, and you can listen in this Chinese manner, you will be giving him/her a great gift. Listen with your heart, with respect and empathy, with your ears and eyes focused on that person. Here are some suggestions of questions or statements:

- How are you TODAY?
- Do you feel the need TODAY/NOW to tell me how you are, or would you rather not right now?
  (Don't conclude here that he/she will NEVER want to talk about it if he/she doesn't want to today)
- I admire your strength but I can also imagine that you sometimes don't feel so strong at all.
- I don't really know what to say and I'm so afraid to say the wrong thing that I notice I don't say anything anymore and I avoid you. That's actually the last thing I want to do.
- Will you please let me know if I say the wrong thing or something that is painful and not properly thought-through?

Choosing to terminate a desired pregnancy

Parents who decide, for medical or personal reasons, to terminate a pregnancy often wrestle with intense emotions of relief as well as grief: relief that their baby and their family will be spared a possible path of suffering, and also grief because they will miss this much-desired baby. Most parents feel that they didn't have a "real" choice, but had to make a heart-wrenching decision between two evils. Above all, most parents feel that they have to defend their decision to terminate the pregnancy. Sometimes they are called to account by those closest to them. It seems they should not be allowed to feel sorrow, or they are marginalised because their baby's death was not spontaneous. Sometimes parents don't agree on the decision: one parent wants to continue the pregnancy and allow their baby to be born, while the other wants to terminate it. Parents can be hurled back and forth between the two choices. Differences of opinion can put pressure on the relationship, in a period where painful decisions need to be taken; decisions that you really don't want to have to take. You need each other more than ever at this distressing time. Heart-wrenching decisions cause heart-wrenching emotions to surface, and that makes it difficult for the parents to see each other's point of view objectively and to listen to feelings and considerations. In most hospitals it's possible to receive guidance from a therapist or social worker to help you make such a distressing decision with its life-long consequences. Once parents have decided to terminate a pregnancy, it can help to have contact with others who have been on a similar path, by talking, chatting online or emailing.

A new pregnancy

Losing a child is a very distressing event. Nevertheless, many parents say afterwards that they discovered new aspects of themselves and each other during that time, such as resilience, perseverance, vulnerability and – however paradoxical it may sound – thankfulness and optimism, hope and trust. They learned new skills and found other ways to communicate. Unfortunately, some friendships are lost but precious new friendships are forged. Grieving parents might dare to do things that they previously never would have thought were possible. Their relationships with family members and friends become more lasting and profound because of the loss. Surviving your loss and then carrying on with your life doesn't mean you've forgotten your child. It means that you've given your baby a place in your new life – life after his/her birth and death. The good days will be more frequent than the bad ones. The loss can be so painful that you might decide never to become pregnant again. You fear that you won't be able to handle the pain of another loss, and your deceased baby cannot of course be replaced. No one can take that unique place. But you won't get your baby back by shutting yourself off from life. Some parents realise only years later that they "stopped living" when they lost their baby. Often they also lose each other because each one grieved in his/her own way. If you have a relapse in your recovery process, don't think you're back to square one. Losing one goal doesn't mean you've lost the whole match. It's completely normal to occasionally be submerged again in the circle of sorrow. It's also completely normal to be extra sad around the anniversary of your baby's birth and/or death. This is called the "anniversary effect". Your body remembers the loss, sometimes even before your mind is aware of it. Learning to live with loss takes time – a lot of time. Nobody can predict how long it will take for you. A mourning period is not finished, by definition, after 12 months have passed. And time doesn't heal all wounds. It's your mourning period and it's only over once you decide it is. You and your partner must decide if and when there is space in your lives and your hearts for a new pregnancy, just as other parents decide when they're ready for a second, third or fourth baby. The new pregnancy following a loss, however, will be different from a "normal" new pregnancy.

Caroline's

STORY

When I was pregnant with my third child, we decided at the beginning to test the baby for Down's syndrome and other birth defects, as I was already 38 years old. When the 12-week ultrasound showed an increased nuchal translucency (fluid in the neck fold), we "chose" to have an amniocentesis. I put "chose" in inverted commas because you actually have little choice. The risk is higher so you want to know what's going on. The amniocentesis revealed that our baby had Down's syndrome and we "chose" to terminate the pregnancy. Again, I've used inverted commas, because that is a choice that's inhuman. We made the decision with our two daughters in mind, because a disabled younger brother would change their lives dramatically. We are older parents and in time they would take over the care of their brother. Yes... we had found out that we were expecting a boy and we wanted him so badly...
We decided at that moment not to tell our daughters about the pregnancy and its termination. It was difficult to keep such intense sorrow secret, but, at the time it seemed like the best way to protect our sensitive small daughters.

The evening before the termination I had to take a pill to soften my uterus. After dinner, while the children were still running about, I took the pill and withdrew to my room. I lay on my bed with a soft toy held tight against me. I was planning to put that toy in our son's coffin. I put my hands on my belly and spoke to my son. I explained our decision to him and asked him to understand that choice. I told him how much we loved him and that he would always be our son, and that we would never forget him. I prayed that I would have a miscarriage that night so that I wouldn't have to be the one to "execute judgement"

on him. The following day we had many important decisions
to think about. Did we want to hold our child and give him a
name? Did we want him to be buried or cremated and did we
want to do this ourselves or rather have the hospital do it?
They were terribly difficult and distressing choices, because we
only had one chance to get it right. After a beautiful delivery,
our son was born. How tiny he was, just 160 grammes. How
beautiful he was – complete. He had perfect little hands and
feet. His mouth was slightly open, worn out from the struggle
he had just faced. I held him until late into the evening. We
named him Phillippe. I'm so grateful to my son that I could
carry him in my womb and feel his first tiny movements. They
had made me so intensely happy, even though it was for just
a short time. I am and will always be his mother and he is and
will always be my son. Our son now has a beautiful grave in a
field with other babies, which we visit regularly.

After a few weeks, my work doctor put pressure on me to
return to work. My husband had gone back after a week. Life
went on as usual; our son was hardly spoken of. Our daughters
didn't even know of his existence. I noticed that I dealt with
the situation very differently from my husband. I wanted to
talk about it a lot while he preferred not to. A few months later,
I noticed I was increasingly sensitive. The GP referred me for
psychological help but I had to wait six months before they
could see me. It felt good to be able to tell my story again, but
unfortunately the psychologist I met was only there for an
initial talk. I had to wait for someone else to have space for me.
I didn't "click" with the psychologist I ended up with and
I stopped going after a couple of sessions.

Then I got pregnant again. The people close to me said the
strangest things, probably well intentioned, but still hurtful:
*"Why was I so upset when the termination had been our
choice?"*, or that we *"could just enjoy this pregnancy now"*, etc.
Unfortunately, the 12-week scan revealed birth defects in this
pregnancy too. That's when I went to see a coach. In the first

session all I could do was cry: such sorrow, so many emotions. I had kept my sadness to myself for too long. I hadn't wanted to bother anyone with it and had received a few blows from painful comments. Not only did I still miss my son, I was very anxious in this fourth pregnancy: afraid to lose another child, but also that something would happen to my two elder daughters. I learned that my feelings were part of the grieving process and that I had the right to grieve, even though it had been my decision to terminate my pregnancy. It felt good to take the time to think about Phillippe during the sessions. I slowly started to accept that it had gone that way; that it was real. The sense of loss became manageable.

The worst moment of the birth for me was when I had to take the pill that set off the procedure. It felt as though I was murdering my son by taking the pill. The coach explained that the pill just served to prepare the uterus for the birth the following day and that there was no way I could have killed my baby with that pill. What a relief! I "replayed" the birth in a special exercise and that had an impact on the way my body felt. I visualised my labour starting spontaneously and our son being born very calmly. We had all the time we wanted to say goodbye to him, and our family and daughters were there to see him and say goodbye. There was such a difference between this version and the loneliness I had felt at the time of his actual birth. I cried with relief and felt much lighter when I left.

In another session I mentioned that I hardly spoke to my husband about our son. We had agreed that we wouldn't tell our daughters anything, to protect them, but that didn't feel right for me anymore. I wanted to respect my husband's feelings and the agreement we had made, but I thought it was awful that the girls didn't know about their brother's existence. The coach gave me the task of sharing my feelings with my husband through a letter. What a tough assignment! I wrote to him about the way my feelings had changed and how much I wanted to tell the girls about their baby brother. I would never have been able to say it to him directly because the emotions were so strong in me. I gave the letter to my husband and went out to the playground with the girls. When we returned, my husband was standing at the door, his eyes red and swollen from crying. He had been doing what he thought was best for me by not talking about our son anymore. I had thought I was doing the best for him by respecting the agreement we had made just before the birth. In the meantime, it hadn't felt right for either of us, but we assumed we knew how the other felt, rather than actually asking: "How do you feel? What are you thinking? Have your feelings changed? Do you miss him as much as I do?"

We told our daughters together about their little brother and they reacted with sadness but also pleasure: *"Mummy, how great that we have a baby brother, but what a shame that he's now in heaven."* It feels so good not to have any secrets from the children anymore. We can now share the sadness between the four of us and our son has become part of the family. We regularly go all together to visit his grave. My sweet little girls decorate his grave each time with something different. On the day Phillippe would have turned one year old they made drawings for him, which they tied to balloons so that they could fly up to him in heaven. I now feel liberated from my guilt towards my son. This has given me more space to think about him and to love him. I feel more relaxed and am less irritable. I also sleep better and can concentrate better at work. My husband and I are back on the same wavelength and spend an evening together at least once a month. When we do that, we ask each other how we're doing instead of presuming we know the answer already. Now that I speak more openly about my loss, people around me spontaneously tell me about their own experiences of loss. This has enabled me to have a completely different connection with some people. Unfortunately, we also lost some friends who couldn't bring themselves to understand our sadness and loss, but so be it. I also learned to literally make room for my sadness. I had had a sort of "ball of sorrow" in my stomach and was given the task of "clearing out" that ball to literally make room for the new little person growing inside me. I faithfully did my relaxation exercises every day and this let me make contact more and more with the new baby. After we heard that the results of the amniocentesis were good, I carefully began to enjoy this fourth pregnancy.

I made a book of memories. At first we hesitated to show photos of Phillippe to our daughters, family members and friends, but he's a part of our family now. I'm proud of the book and it brings me comfort. It feels like Phillippe also has a "baby book". A year after Phillippe, we had a third daughter, our fourth child, who is just as desired and welcome as the first three.

Lisa's

STORY

At the start of my second pregnancy I had a throat infection that was so bad I needed antibiotics, and since then had felt unwell. I also caught a bad stomach flu and regularly had fever. When I was 20 weeks pregnant I suddenly started bleeding, due to a low-lying placenta. After spending 24 hours in hospital I was allowed home and stopped working on the advice of the gynaecologist. Two weeks later I had (a lot of) blood loss again and was admitted to hospital. Since our baby wasn't yet old enough to survive outside of the womb, we were sent to the teaching hospital. I can't describe what that does to you. You alternate between being listless, needy and aggressive. You keep extending your boundaries: you have no control anymore over your own life and after a while this seems normal to you. For example, when you finally get to sleep, someone will come and wake you up for a shot or a pill. You also attach enormous value to a "look in the eye" or casual remarks made by doctors and nurses.

I often felt that I wasn't being taken seriously, as if the doctors and nurses knew better than I did what was happening in my body, and as if I wasn't mentally competent to make my own decisions. When I got a fever again, the doctors didn't know why. The antibiotics I was given didn't work. I had dreadful headaches as well as Braxton Hicks contractions, cramps that felt like contractions, but, according to the doctors, were not. One time I had a sort of fever fit, a very cold shivering episode that lasted half an hour and made me really afraid I was going to die. It was a shock reaction to the antibiotics.

Ten days after being admitted to the teaching hospital I felt fluid leaking and feared my waters had broken. The nurse didn't think so – again I felt I wasn't being taken seriously. Later that day it turned out my waters had broken and there was hardly any amniotic fluid left. The baby was in the least convenient position, with one foot down, one knee pulled up and the umbilical cord in between, under his bottom, as if he was riding the umbilical cord. I was also losing a lot of blood and blood clots. The iron in my blood sank in a couple of days by one point and the infection measurements were sky high.

I was 24 weeks and four days pregnant. When I was admitted I had been told that from 24 weeks our child had a chance of survival outside the womb. I was fully aware that he had just a tiny chance if he were to be born now, but still: he had a chance. Two days later, I felt something come out of me. It was the umbilical cord. Amid panic I was taken to the delivery room. My husband and my mother were with me. The contractions started. Because I had been using blood thinners for several weeks, I wasn't allowed an epidural. Fairly soon I got the urge to push, but wasn't allowed to because the baby was in the breech position. I wasn't dilated enough. The doctors were worried his head would get stuck in the uterus. It was almost impossible to fight the pushing contractions. They told me a foot was born. To make matters worse it seems our son had lifted his arms up, as if calling for help. His arms were by his head, expanding the head width and making it even more difficult for him to be born. There were so many people around my bed, including an entire paediatric team, ready to take over. The gynaecologist began pulling on my baby. I was so scared at that moment; I thought they were going to rip him apart. I was in so much pain and kept screaming: *"STOP! STOP!"* But they didn't stop. *"We can't stop now,"* they said. The pain was unbearable; my thoughts were all over the place. *"I want to keep him inside my body, now, in me, he's still alive."* And at the same time: *"I have to let him go, he has a better chance of survival on the outside."*

Gabriel was born and they laid him on my stomach. They
assumed that he had not survived the horrifying delivery with
all that pulling. My husband noticed that Gabriel was breathing
and notified the paediatrician. The latter found a heartbeat of
60 beats per minute. "There's a heartbeat, I'm taking him."

My mother went with Gabriel and the doctor while my
husband stayed with me. I lay there, with empty arms and
an empty belly, alternating again between hope and dread.
It seemed to last an eternity and at the same time, time was
standing still. Nobody could tell me anything. The bubble I had
been in for the last few weeks was a sort of bad film with this
moment as its lowest point. I wasn't completely there. It was
all to much to take in. I was entirely preoccupied with myself
– wondering how and why I had ended up in this horror film.

Half an hour later the paediatrician came back with a bundle
in his arms. Without asking, he laid Gabriel, swaddled, on my
stomach. His heart was still beating but he wasn't going to
make it. Gabriel looked a bit alarming– more like a frightening
old grandpa with lots of frown marks on his forehead than a
little baby. I could see how he had battled, how much he was
suffering. It didn't feel like he was my child. I would have
preferred not to have him lying on my stomach. But he still lay
there. It felt surreal. It was at least half an hour before his heart
finally stopped beating. I saw how lovingly my husband looked
at Gabriel, but I couldn't find anything to love in him. I even
regretted that we had "wasted" the name Gabriel on this child.
We couldn't use it again if we had another boy. The doctors and
nurses advised me to take him home with me. I really didn't
want to do that either. I let my husband convince me. Once
we were home, we laid Gabriel in the baby room. I focused my
attention on our eldest daughter, Katie. I couldn't bring myself
to face Gabriel.

The hospital immediately offered me psychological support.
I'm a very practical-minded person and not much of a talker
and I just wanted to forget the whole episode as quickly as

possible. It wasn't going to bring Gabriel back anyway. Instead of talking about Gabriel's birth, I chose to use the EMDR session (see Chapter 7) to talk to the psychologist about the birth of my elder daughter. I found that easier. *"That's okay,"* the psychologist said. I didn't need the sessions anymore after a few months. I felt I had more or less said everything I needed to say. I had done what I had to do. I looked after our daughter, went to work and to birthday parties, but I didn't feel anything. I was like a zombie. Six months later, my husband wanted us to try for another baby, but I couldn't bear the thought of it. Gradually things went downhill with me. My work was suffering: I couldn't concentrate and was tetchy. My relationship with my husband was rocky. I retreated further into my shell when my husband tried to get me to do "something fun" and meet up with our friends. He clearly meant it well, he wanted to pull me out of my negative spiral, I see that now, but I had no desire for social gatherings. Nothing really felt "fun" anymore. I hardly slept – just a couple of hours a night. The tiredness made the vicious circle complete.

Almost a year after Gabriel was born, I went to see a coach. In the very first session she asked me about Gabriel and whether I had photos of him. She was the first healthcare provider who had called him by his name and shown an interest in him. I took a photo album along to the next session, as well as a diary that my mother had put together of my stay at the hospital and Gabriel's birth. I hadn't yet been able to read the whole of the diary and I could barely look at the photos. We did that together with the coach. What a beautiful gift it had been from my mother to have made that diary! Step by step, we walked through the entire hospital episode and discussed how and why I felt the way I did. I could finally bring myself to look at the pictures taken during the birth. The coach explained how you could see from the marks on Gabriel's neck how his head had stayed stuck in the uterus while his legs were already born. She drew my attention to the bruises on his legs from where the doctor had pulled hard to try to get him out.

She asked me to choose the best picture of Gabriel and to describe what I liked about it. I chose one that was taken an hour after he had died. His face on the photo was smooth; the battle that he had fought was less visible. He even seemed peaceful: much better than that tiny wrinkled and anguished old man that they had laid on my belly to die. It was as if I was able to meet him again for the first time. I started to recognise features in him of my husband, myself and our elder daughter. The longer I looked at the photo, the more Gabriel became "mine". I think I must have sat looking at that photo for an hour.

I had had EMDR with the psychologist just after Gabriel's birth, but, almost a year later, I still had symptoms. The coach suggested I try EMDR again. She asked which image I most avoided thinking about. That was the one of the paediatrician bringing Gabriel all wrapped-up to place him on my belly. I first thought that this scene was the worst for me because I was ashamed that my son frightened me. But by seeing the situation again before me, I suddenly realised what I had suppressed all this time. Just after he was born, Gabriel lay on my stomach, just as his elder sister had when she was just born, and that felt okay. Then my husband saw that Gabriel was breathing, the paediatrician heard there was a heartbeat and took him away. I thought they were going to make him "better" again.

It was only when I saw Gabriel's frowning face and heard the doctor say he wasn't going to make it that I realised they were bringing him to me to die. That was so not what I wanted! And that's why I didn't want him lying on my stomach. The pain was just too great. The only way I could deal with the pain was to reject my darling Gabriel.

The EMDR session brought to the surface my helplessness, powerlessness, the pain and horror, my need to run away and my rejection of Gabriel. I also saw why I hadn't wanted to take him home with me. I wanted a living Gabriel in the cot and

I resented my husband for being so enthusiastic about this dead Gabriel. He had accepted this Gabriel completely, while I wanted as little as possible to do with him because he was dead. It sounds awful, but I was disgusted by this dead Gabriel and disgusted with myself for feeling that disgust. He was my baby boy. What kind of mother feels disgust for her child? I felt so guilty when I said those words. My coach helped me to understand that my feeling of disgust was probably a shock reaction – the shock was so overwhelming that I just wanted to run out of the delivery room. My disgust was not aimed at Gabriel but at the whole situation, the fact that the child we wanted so much was going to die, in spite of my having done my absolute best for weeks to keep him alive. I immediately felt less guilty: I was disgusted with the situation, not with Gabriel. What a liberating thought.

The story now made sense; I finally understood what had happened and why I had reacted like that. I had actually been paralysed by fear. I couldn't understand what was happening and I didn't want it to happen. Gabriel had been safe inside my body all that time. I had fought for him all those weeks I was in the hospital. After he was born I couldn't make sure he was safe anymore... and he died. In the following sessions I "overwrote" the upsetting memories of the birth using a special technique. I could say how I wanted Gabriel to have been born and how I wanted to have said goodbye to him. That exercise was beautiful and gave me peace. In my version, I gave birth in my own trusted hospital with my own gynaecologist present at the birth. Gabriel was born serenely, without any pushing or pulling. There was no panic among the medical team. He was laid on my stomach, I saw for myself that he wasn't breathing. My husband held us both. The doctors and nurses left the room. Gabriel died on my stomach. There was no frown on his face, no visible suffering, it was peaceful and calm. My husband and I were with him. There was no paediatrician, no ceremony. We experienced Gabriel's birth together. I was even able to admire Gabriel while I visualised him on my stomach. I could actually feel him lying there. I pictured that one good photo in front of me. What a gift, in spite of the sad ending. This time, it did feel good to take Gabriel home with us. I was finally proud of him and of myself, more than a year after his birth and death.

It's now two years down the line and although I don't think I will ever be able to fully process such a traumatic event, I can find a place for it. Things are going well at work and also between my husband and me. Our third child took a long time to make an appearance. Eighteen months after Gabriel, I had a miscarriage. My husband and I underwent that sad episode together. I will never again have a care-free pregnancy, but in the meantime, I gave birth to our third child, Sara, a beautiful baby girl. Her birth and early infancy were simultaneously a highly emotional and very happy time. Our sorrow for Gabriel is real and we can embrace it, next to the joy we have from our two other children. I'm thankful that Gabriel, our second child and first son, now really has a place in my family and in my life.

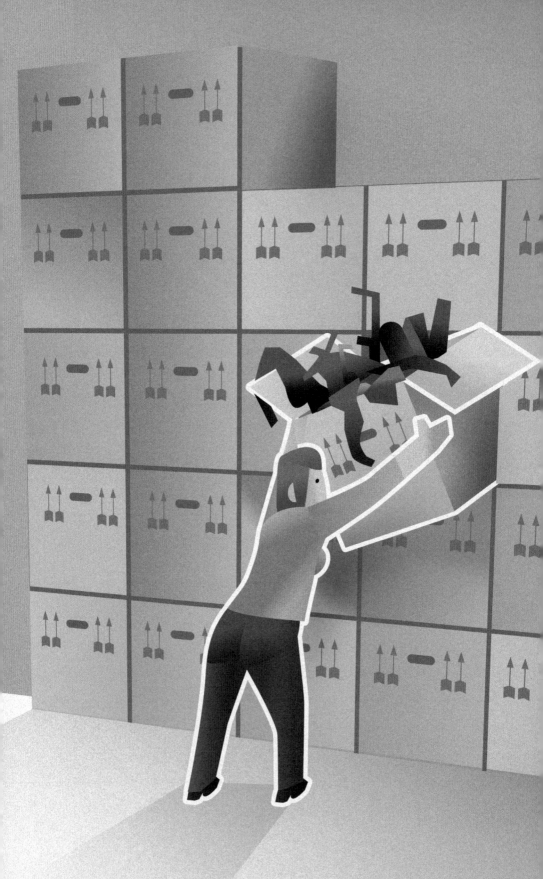

CHAPTER 7

Treating post-traumatic stress complaints following childbirth

As we've seen in the previous chapters, traumatic birth experiences are still considered a taboo subject, and I hope this book will help to break that. The taboo is upheld partly because women don't easily express how big a role their distressing birth experience plays in their lives, and partly because PTSD symptoms, such as concentration problems and irritability, are too often ascribed to "hormones". PTSD symptoms are also not identified often enough by health professionals because they overlap with "normal" pregnancy and postpartum complaints, or are confused with postpartum depression. In addition, not all health professionals concerned with childbirth are aware that a traumatic birth can lead to PTSD complaints, and that these complaints can be treated (relatively easily). A traumatic event sets off a dysfunctional neural network (fear memory) in your brain. If you don't do anything about it, the network remains, with repercussions for you, your baby and your relationship.

Neural network

It's impossible for your brain to remember everything that happens to you in the day, as there are far too many stimuli in each day. The more impact an event has on you, the greater the neural activity it triggers in your brain. The event is stored as a memory and a new neural network is formed: an image or series of images are connected like a film to thoughts about yourself and emotions/feelings that you associate with that film. It can be a neural network of positive associations, but also negative ones. The more threatening the situation that you experienced is, the more the brain wants to store it, to prevent you from getting into such a frightening situation again or to help you recognise it in the future so that you can save yourself. After you've been bitten once by a dog, you're extra careful around dogs. A neural network has formed in your brain: the image of a dog barking and running towards you with uncovered teeth. You've connected this image to a thought: get help, danger, this dog is going to hurt me, and to an emotion: in this case, usually fear. The more negative experiences you have with dogs, the more fearful you will be of them. Your brain gives a lot of weight to this neural network in order to protect you from further danger. The more negatively you interpret the event, the more negative thoughts and feelings you have about yourself, the greater the "danger triangle" (see Chapter 2) your brain uses to mark this experience. For your birth experience, this danger triangle will be activated every time you walk back into the hospital, or if you get pregnant again. If an anxious person is put into a brain scanner and asked to think back to the negative event, you see that the same parts of their brain are activated as during the actual event. This happens for negative as well as positive events. You can use this to let high-level athletes visualise a start or a match. This activates the same parts of the brain as a real match. I will come back to this when I talk about preparing to give birth again (see Chapter 9), where you can use this to your advantage.

"With hindsight I realise that I was paralysed with fear during the birth of our second child because I hadn't processed the distressing birth of our eldest daughter. That time, the gynaecologist had stormed into the delivery room, his coat flapping, barely introducing himself. He pushed the very young assistant to the side, shoved the ventouse inside me, made a cut, pulled my baby out and left again. I felt completely besieged by the experience, but let myself be distracted by our baby daughter, Sara, who made it all seem worthwhile. It's not for nothing that they say that you forget how distressing childbirth is. I focused on Sara and on the breastfeeding and soon forgot the unpleasantness of the birth... until I got pregnant with our second child. I pushed away the thoughts about the upcoming birth for as long as I could. I was too busy for pregnancy yoga and 'had to' help organise my friend's wedding just before my maternity leave started. It was during my maternity leave that I realised that I couldn't escape the birth. I started having nightmares, which woke me up bathed in sweat, my heart pounding. After that I would stare at the ceiling for an hour, unable to move from fear.

When the midwife asked if I had made a birth plan, I replied that I didn't believe in birth plans since my last experience, because nothing then had gone according to plan. The second time, my labour began with my waters breaking, but there were no contractions. The next day the birth was induced. It all went so fast that there was no time to do anything about the pain. I had a feeling I was outside of my body, looking down at myself from the ceiling: an empty shell giving birth, nodding, breathing, but absent. The baby's heart rate dropped to a precarious level. Once again, they needed to use the ventouse. Luckily, this time I was surrounded by the kindest medical staff. Afterwards, I felt bad that I had ignored the distress of my first birth experience for so long. Doing that had left me completely unprepared for my second birth. If only I had known about EMDR beforehand, if only someone had seen through my brave act when I spoke of my first birth and my laconic stance towards my second birth... If only, if only... I'm sure I would have had a chance to push my second baby out without help.

I had two EMDR sessions, one to process the first birth and one for the second. What surprised me was that the same method was used each time, but the two sessions played out very differently. Now I look back on two intense experiences, but without any guilt or other unpleasantness. If we ever decide to try for a third child, I'll go back to my coach to help me prepare myself for the birth."
(Aygul, 27 years old)

> If your body stays in a state of stress – even after the birth – and if you remain hypervigilant, you can find yourself in a vicious circle: from tense, to overstrained, to burned-out. To be continuously under pressure exhausts you both physically and mentally. Your nerves are continuously raw and are therefore much more quickly overstimulated. Your immune system is weakened, making you more vulnerable to infections. Your

digestive system, powers of thought and concentration become secondary, giving you physical and psychological complaints. If you don't break through this negative circle there may be depression and/or a burnout looming just around the corner. These force your body and mind to rest. EMDR *(Eye Movement Desensitization and Reprocessing)* can help you process a disturbing birth experience.

The origins of EMDR

When out for a walk in 1987, psychologist Francine Shapiro was ambushed by a disturbing memory. Coincidentally, while it happened, she looked quickly a few times from left to right and noticed that the emotional impact of the memory was reduced. She felt that the rapid eye movements somehow helped her to neutralise the memory. She began by testing out her theory on her friends, with tantalising results. After that, she examined whether her "eye movement technique" could also help her clients process traumatic experiences. This turned out to be the case, including for Vietnam War veterans whom she had been treating for a long time – without much success – for Post-Traumatic Stress Disorder (PTSD). Two years later (in 1989), Shapiro published on her procedure (which she had standardised by then, and named EMDR).

EMDR is the "gold standard" for treating trauma

Since then there has been more than enough scientific evidence that EMDR is effective, but exactly how it works is still unclear. In 2012 the Trimbos Institute (Netherlands Institute for Mental Health and Addiction) updated the multidisciplinary guideline for anxiety disorders and PTSD for the second time. In this guideline, EMDR and cognitive behavioural therapy (CBT, see Chapter 8) are seen as the "gold standard" for the treatment of PTSD symptoms.

Despite this, EMDR is (unfortunately) not yet the standard therapy for processing traumatic birth experiences, and traumatic birth experiences are still given insufficient recognition by health professionals and by society.

Chapter 2 offers two definitions of trauma. The dictionary definition is *"a physical or psychological wound, caused by an accident, operation or distressing life event"*. According to the Diagnostic and Statistical Manual of Mental Disorders (DSM-5), in order to diagnose PTSD there must be *"actual or threatened death, serious injury and/or sexual violation"*. For ease of use we can call the first definition "trauma with a small t" and the second "Trauma with a capital T". The majority of traumatic birth experiences fall within the first category.

I believe that these traumas with a small t also merit recognition and treatment, especially considering the impact of untreated trauma on a woman, her child and her relationship with her partner (see Chapters 3, 4 and 5). For this reason I've been using EMDR, since 2010, to help clients process their traumatic births. There have been some pilot studies on the effectiveness of EMDR for processing traumatic births. Gynaecologist Claire Stramrood shook the world of childbirth care awake with her PhD research on *Post-Traumatic Stress following pregnancy and childbirth*. I'm very proud that my practice-based knowledge has been corroborated by Stramrood's scientific research. At the moment, research is being carried out in the *Onze Lieve Vrouwe hospital* in Amsterdam on employing EMDR during pregnancy for women who have PTSD symptoms resulting from an earlier birth experience, or women who have extreme anxiety about their upcoming first birth. The results of this *OptiMUM* study are expected in 2017.

The goal of EMDR

EMDR therapy has two important objectives: to reduce fear, and to make the patient think in a different way about a traumatic experience, thus reducing PTSD symptoms.

1. **Reducing fear:** A traumatic birth experience can make you unduly anxious. EMDR helps to restore balance. If you see the whole birth as a film, during the EMDR session you pause the film on the scene that you find most upsetting at that moment. This is called the worst image, target or initial image. It can be another part of the birth than the one you found to be the worst before (during or just after the birth). The EMDR therapist asks about the tension you feel in your body when you bring to mind that worst image. You score the tension you feel on a scale from zero to ten, where ten is the highest possible amount of tension, and zero is no tension at all. Most women give their tension a value of eight or higher when they're thinking about their worst memory of the birth. During the EMDR session, the tension level will be brought to a minimum, i.e. from eight (or higher) to zero. For many women this is hard to believe, because they have been carrying this tension for many months or even years. Believe it or not, at the end of the EMDR session(s) you will be able to recall the worst memory without being rigid with stress, bursting into tears or having a nervous breakdown.

2. **Changing the meaning** you give to your experience (cognitive restructuring): Following EMDR treatment, women think differently (more neutrally) about their distressing birth experience. This is called cognitive restructuring. This is why the R for Reprocessing was added to the EMDR method. After having EMDR you're able to separate your upsetting memories of the birth (in the past) from the fact that you are safe in the present. In Chapter 2 I use the metaphor of being struck by lightning during childbirth. If the "lightning" is still in your system, your alarm system will be set to extra sensitive. The smallest

thing will launch you into fight-or-flight mode. Psychologists call this hyper-arousal, meaning that you are overly alert to all sorts of stimuli. EMDR can help you remove the lightning from your system. During the treatment you focus your attention on a distracting stimulus of following the therapist's fingers with your eyes (or listening to beeps through headphones), and this brings the hyper-arousal down to a normal level. Because the stimulus (the moving fingers) is repetitive, the situation feels increasingly familiar and safe in the here and now. Your brain gives a new meaning to the frightening experience, and you are able to recall it in a more neutral manner.

"I first thought that the worst part of the birth was when the baby's heart rate dropped and that that was why I was so anxious that something was going to happen to Evie. I checked at least ten times a night to see if she was still breathing.

During the EMDR session, I realised that what I had found the most disturbing was the presence of a student midwife (without my permission). I felt the student's hesitation during the delivery and that made me unsure of myself. The fact that the heart rate fell before the baby was born was frightening, but the fear that I saw in the student's eyes was much, much worse. That moment seemed to last for an hour: Evie's slow heartbeat, the way the student looked questioningly at me and at the midwife, who just stood there and looked questioningly back at her. I understand that the midwife wanted to give the student the chance to make a decision, but at that moment all that was going through my mind was that my baby was going to die because I didn't have the courage to speak out and guard my borders, because I was so desperate for their approval. During the EMDR session I could feel my heart beating in my throat when I relived that frozen moment. I felt powerless, helpless, afraid and sad all at the same time. I was furious with myself for not speaking up and not saying that I didn't want a student at my birth. I was angry with the midwife for not asking my permission beforehand and because she stood there without intervening, whereas she had promised she would take action if it became necessary. I was mad at the student for being so unsure, and I was disappointed in myself because her insecurity had wiped away my own self-confidence. And I was afraid because I could see her fear and saw that she didn't know what to do. If she didn't know what I needed to do and the midwife didn't say or do anything, how was I to know what to do? The EMDR made me re-experience all of this, sort of simultaneously as well as consecutively – very strange – as if time was standing still and also going around in circles. After about an hour I could look at the image and the heart rate drop was a lot less frightening. It was as if I was watching a senseless film. The facial expressions of the student and the midwife had also vanished, or faded. I saw myself lying there and I thought: okay, now you have to do it yourself, you can do it. And then I pushed my daughter out. I went automatically from the negative thought *'I'm failing/I can't do this'* to the positive thought *'I can do this'* and the feeling followed suit. Before the EMDR, I found I was 'not okay' and neither were the student or the midwife. My coach asked if my need to be "nice:" also affected other aspects of my life. Well, yes... I have it in pretty much all aspects of my life! Strangely enough, the EMDR also changed things for me in that respect. Whenever possible, I stop everything and take time during stressful events to ask myself, what do I want? I regularly ask for time to think so that I can decide what I want and how I want it. This helps me protect my boundaries much better, including at work. I had always thought that people wouldn't like me if I did that, but I'm being told now that they like the fact that I'm more clear about my needs.

Since the EMDR I'm also much less over-anxious with regard to Evie. I decided that I saved her life when nobody else was doing anything and that she was perfectly capable of overcoming the birth and the slow heart rate, so we can both rely on ourselves and each other. I'm okay, Evie is okay and the midwives are also okay. I now understand that that frozen moment gave me a distorted image of the midwife and the student. It probably only lasted a minute at the most and I'm sure the midwife would have taken over." (Marjory, 31 years old)

There is enough evidence that EMDR works and there are a number of (partially conflicting) hypotheses about how it works exactly. The most plausible theory at the moment is the working memory taxation theory.

The working memory taxation theory

Your memory consists of three different parts:

- **The sensory memory:** This stores all the information received through your senses: images, sounds, smells, tastes and textures that you have touched. Your sensory memory works as a sort of filter that passes information on to your working memory. The storage capacity of the sensory memory is very large but you process most sensory stimuli unconsciously. Your brain stores them with a thin thread leading to the corresponding event, thoughts and feelings. The more thoughts and feelings there are connected to a particular smell or taste, the more important it is for your brain to remember the event, and the more storage capacity and labels that memory will be given in your mind. If you then come across that particular smell again (for example, the smell of disinfectant in a hospital), see that image again (when walking into the lobby of the hospital), or hear that sound (the beeps of the CTG device on your friend's birth video), the corresponding event (your birth experience) will be recalled from your memory. Recalling it in this way is just like being back in the middle of the original experience.
- **The working memory** (short-term memory): With your working memory, you process the information that comes in. Picture your working memory as a shipment or post room. All the information (post) comes in and you must decide which post box in the long-term memory each letter needs to go into. If you picture your long-term memory as a complex supercomputer, the working memory, in comparison, is like a simple, old-fashioned counting frame. Luckily, the counting frame and the supercomputer work very well together in your brain.
- **The long-term memory:** This is where all your memories are stored. The more impression an experience or event (such as your distressing birth) has had on you and the more intense the emotion you felt during the event, the greater the storage capacity and danger triangles that event will have in your memory. A high-impact experience is linked to other, earlier

experiences and a new neural network is formed. The more frequently certain information comes back and the more associations there are with an event or a thought pattern, the better you will remember it. That event or thought pattern is then easily accessible in your memory.

Adaptive Information Processing (AIP)

Shapiro's theory is that people have an information processing system *(Adaptive Information Processing or AIP)*, that intuitively helps process and heal traumatic memories. Your brain wants to restore the balance, just as your body is always trying to restore balance. If, for example, you've drunk a lot of tea, you have more liquid in your body and will need to go to the toilet more often. If the weather is very warm, you sweat, which cools your body down. Your body is constantly working on maintaining its balance without you even realising it.

The AIP process in your brain can be compared with the way your body heals a cut on your skin. First, the blood platelets stop the bleeding, then a scab forms over the wound and finally the skin heals from the inside. Sometimes, something goes wrong in the healing process and the wound becomes infected. If you keep scratching at a wound, it doesn't get a chance to heal. Unprocessed trauma is stored messily and dysfunctionally, as if you stuffed it into an overfull and bulging packing box. You've been through something intense and your brain needs to "park" the experience quickly, somewhere where the overflowing packing box is out of the way as much as possible. Your brain plans to unpack it later, when you're less stressed, and to store the experience where it belongs, with other experiences in the same category. However, if you stay in a stressed mode, the box will never be cleared away and you risk tripping over it regularly. EMDR can help you clear away that packing box.

Following the therapist's fingers in an EMDR session, you move your eyes from side to side. The eye movement stimulates the brain's adaptive system (AIP). This should allow you to process the information in existing experiences and to integrate memories and store everything in a more functional way.

Note: the existence of such a processing system (AIP) has not yet been scientifically proven. It is one of the hypotheses that could explain why EMDR is so effective.

Description of an EMDR session

During an EMDR session you (briefly) recall the worst moment of your birth experience. The act of calling to mind the memory (opening the packing box and looking to see what's inside), uses a portion of the (limited) capacity of your working memory. The same working memory is simultaneously taxed with a simple task, continuously for about 30 seconds. You follow the moving fingers of or your therapist with your eyes, or listen to beeps through headphones, alternately in your left and right ear. You're standing, in a sense, with one foot in the past (as you relive your upsetting birth) and one foot in the present (because you're safe and relaxed on a chair in your therapist's office).

After 30 seconds of eye movements or beeps, the therapist will ask you what's happening to you inside. There will be thoughts and feelings surfacing, you don't need to do anything about them. Reactions to processing differ from person to person, because each one has had a different birth experience. Sometimes you will encounter images and feelings that don't seem to be connected to the birth. Whatever comes up in your mind is okay, as long as the tension in your body slowly starts to dissipate.

Your EMDR therapist will help you to maintain your complete focus on your upsetting feelings and thoughts throughout the whole session, so that you can follow your own train of thought or associations. I like to use a "train" metaphor to describe the procedure. The train departs from the top of a mountain. The higher the mountain (or tension and emotions), the faster the train will ride. For 30 seconds the train races down the mountain at maximum speed (while the eye movements are taking place), and then pauses at a station (the resting moment when you tell your therapist what's going through you, which images you see and what feelings are surfacing). The train then continues on the same track to the next station, and so on until the track ends. At this point, there is a "track change" at a station and the train continues its journey on new thoughts, images or feelings, until the train has travelled all the possible tracks and comes to a stop – on its own – in the valley. Each train of thought will be followed in this way, repeatedly, until the tension is gone. A new neural network forms, as a result of the EMDR, to replace the old, frightening network (fear memory network). You clear away the overflowing packing box by yourself and place its contents somewhere in your brain where they don't get in the way anymore, where you don't have to trip over them unexpectedly. Clients often say that the images fade or become smaller during the EMDR session.

EMDR is not hypnosis or magic – it's all about focus. You focus your attention on a small, distracting task that distracts your working memory from the disturbing memory. It can be compared to the way illusionists and conjurors distract your thoughts while performing a magic trick. EMDR cannot be compared to hypnosis because that puts you into a different state of consciousness. In an EMDR session, in contrast, you are fully and consciously present in the here and now. EMDR is a powerful and seemingly simple method. Perhaps this is why it has taken so long for the regular world of psychological care to accept this therapy. After an EMDR session I often hear clients exclaim: *"It seems to be gone. It surely can't be that simple, can it?"* But it can be that simple. Your brain wants nothing more than to clear away that irritating messy packing box, and EMDR helps it to do just that. Compared with other psychotherapy methods, there is very little talking in an EMDR session. This is because a lot of talking disturbs your ability to process the trauma. There is currently research into computer games and even an app, which, when used soon after a distressing experience, might prevent or reduce the onset of PTSD symptoms.

"I tried EMDR because I had chronic pain in my C-section scar after giving birth. At the hospital they couldn't find anything; the wound seemed to have healed perfectly. The pain reminded me constantly of my traumatic birth. I couldn't find any information in pregnancy books or hospital brochures, so I looked online. On internet forums I came across stories of women who had suffered chronic pain in their C-section scar or from their episiotomy. A number of these women had found relief from EMDR, so I wanted to try it out. I had no idea what EMDR was exactly. When the coach started waving her fingers in front of my eyes I took some time to get used to it.

I found it hard to keep my head still and the moving fingers made me dizzy. She adjusted the distance between us and also the speed of her movements seemed to be different. Soon I was back in the middle of my birth "film". It was very real, while at the same time it wasn't, as if I were watching it from a distance, watching a tense and sometimes surreal film in which I was playing the main role. My heart was racing and I began to sweat. I started breathing very fast. The coach reminded me that I was now safe in her office and helped me to breathe evenly from my stomach, while she continued to wave her fingers in front of me. I felt like I had been doing some intensive sports without having left my chair. After a while everything felt calmer. The disturbing image became smaller and my vision of myself, watching the film, became larger. At the end I was watching the image with a big grin on my face. I had grown a baby in my tummy and had become a mother. The way in which my son was born felt less important to me after I'd had the EMDR. The pain from the scar has also lessened considerably since then." (Rana, 24 years old)

EMDR therapists

You can ask your GP to refer you to an EMDR therapist. You can ask the EMDR therapist beforehand if they have any experience with processing childbirth trauma

"Just after my first baby was born, I had EMDR sessions with a psychologist at the hospital. Two years later, when I was pregnant again, I found I was short-tempered again and was also very worried about the upcoming delivery. In the end, it appeared that the most upsetting thing for me hadn't been the birth itself, but the gynaecologist's report. I had really had a hellish birth and many things had gone wrong. On the report she had written 'no complications, ventouse extraction due to maternal exhaustion'. No complications?! I had been 'practise pushing' for hours, but the report said I had pushed for just an hour and a half. And... maternal exhaustion? What do you expect after all those hours? And yes, I did beg her to help me. But I meant with support and coaching, not a pump to suck my child out of me. I could have gone on a bit longer if I had been assured that there would be some progress. All the practise pushing that led to nothing made me lose all my courage and determination. What is 'practise pushing', anyway? You either push or you don't! Fifteen minutes of pushing with all my might and then puffing because it wasn't working and then they left me alone to 'wait for the baby to come down further, because he was too high up for the ventouse and too comfortable to justify a C-section'. I really thought I was going to die, and in fact I wanted to die because I felt so lonely and so hopeless every time I was left all by myself.

During the EMDR session I lost all notion of time. It was very intense but also felt wonderful to be able to neutralise the film in one go. It was tough but I felt how the image began to change in my mind; it began to quiver slightly, like the way asphalt looks in very hot weather, as if it could evaporate at any moment. I can't describe it any other way. It actually doesn't matter how I try to describe it, the important thing is that it worked! My coach helped me make a plan for the second birth. I hired a doula to stay with me so that I wouldn't ever have to be alone. My second birth experience was so positive and warm! I felt held, support and nurtured by my partner, the doula, the midwife and the nurse. For this reason, I can't agree with the title of this book, because after a hellish birth, the second one was like heaven. Perfect childbirth is not a myth!" (Elsa, 31 years old)

The FHER method:
Feel it, Heal it, Erase it, Replace it

In Chapter 1 we compare burying emotions with trying to hold a beach ball under water. It's impossible. Your muscles will ache and the beach ball will always win. With a big burst of energy it will fly in a big arc far above the water and then drift calmly away on the surface of the water. After a couple of waves the water will also become calm again. It's such a waste of energy to use all your strength to try to maintain the beach ball of your feelings underwater. *"You've got to feel it to heal it."* Feelings want to be felt. Yes, it really is that simple. And it's so complicated at the same time, because you have taught yourself, out of an instinct of self-preservation, to ignore these feelings. Just try to change this without outside help. EMDR can help you process your disturbing experience and to sort through and clear away the unpacked box. Besides EMDR, I use other methods to help clients to "feel it and heal it". For example, I have an exercise whereby we rewind the videotape of the disturbing film *(erase it)* and record it again *(replace it)*.

I adapted this method from the scientifically proven method of mitigating nightmares by imagining a different ending to your dream during the day. You actively "save" the new ending in your brain by writing down your new dream and reading it before you go to sleep. Within a couple of weeks you will dream the new ending instead of the nightmare. If you would like to read more on this, look up the terms "rescripting", "IRT *(Imagery Rehearsal Treatment)*" or "LDT *(Lucid Dreaming Therapy)*" – or see the Bibliography.

Back to your birth experience: your brain wants nothing more than to heal from the distressing experience. There is the experience that you actually had, but you also had an expectation beforehand of how your (ideal) birth would be. The FHER method allows you to fuse the two together. You erase the upsetting experience and replace it with one that feels right for you. You describe how your labour should have gone. You use all your five senses for this in order to make the situation as real as possible before your eyes: what do you see, feel, smell and hear around you? Who is with you, and what are they doing to support you? I train midwives and doctors, who, in addition to their medical studies, have also completed a coaching training, to become childbirth processing specialists. A number of psychologists have also specialised in this field. A childbirth processing specialist can help you to replace your traumatic birth experience with a neutral or even positive experience.

"When I was a child, my father was the one who cuddled us. My mother was more the type to tell us to 'stop complaining, hold your chin up and keep going'. My father passed away when I was 14. My brother was 28 then and already lived alone. I don't remember ever having been hugged since my father's death.

Giving birth completely overwhelmed me. I'm a 38-year-old single mother by choice. I've wanted to have children for as long as I can remember, but haven't been in a serious relationship since I was 30. When I was 36, I decided to try artificial insemination with the help of a (gay) donor whom I knew. I gave birth five weeks early and after just five hours of labour. It all went so quickly. The friend who was supposed to be at the birth to support me only arrived ten minutes after my son Tony was born. At that point Tony had already been taken away by the paediatrician because he wasn't well. Everybody said how well I had done, but I hardly knew what had happened to me. My baby was unwell and all my attention was on him. He was so fragile that I wasn't allowed to cuddle him. I was only allowed to stroke his hand through the incubator. It all seemed so surreal and overwhelming.

When I found myself in a state of depression, I was referred to a specialised coach: a childbirth processing specialist. When she asked me how I had experienced the birth, I said it had all gone much too fast to really experience it. It happened in a flash and the period after it had been so much more stressful than the birth itself because of the worries surrounding Tony's health. She noticed that I put my arms on my shoulders while I told my story, as if I was giving myself a hug. She asked if I needed a hug. I burst into tears and couldn't stop crying. Sorrow and loss were the central themes of our discussions after that. Since my father's death I had largely buried my feelings. Missing my father, his comforting hugs, missing a partner and being touched by a loved one, the stress of the ultra-quick delivery and my dread of losing Tony as well – I suddenly saw how it was all connected. I had kept shutting myself off from intense feelings so that I could stay on my feet, when my father died, just as when Tony was born. I learned to feel my feelings and to listen to them, to hug and support myself. I also learned to call a friend when all the powerful emotions seemed to engulf me. Twenty years after his death, I cried for my father as if he had died the day before. It felt as though the depression was a lump of coagulated sorrow that was now coming out.

It was a very difficult period for me, and for one month Tony went every day to the crèche because I was incapable of looking after him. I had my hands full just caring for myself. Slowly, I went from feeling it to healing it. I had EMDR treatment for the fast birth and the distressing postnatal period and after that I used FHER to rescript the birth. I rewound the original videotape of Tony's birth and rerecorded my ideal delivery on to the same tape, over the upsetting version. In my ideal version, I gave birth calmly at home, a day after my due date and this time my friend was with me. Bizarrely, I then had a strong desire for the sperm donor to be present at the birth too. Only then did the birth feel complete, intimate and profound. It was a beautiful experience.

When I now recall the birth, I know how it happened (in reality) but I have connected it to the pleasant feeling of the second 'birth' that I visualised together with my coach. It's very strange and hard to put into words, but for me, the two experiences have now melted into one. To seal the whole experience, I had a bath together with Tony. That was such a wonderful feeling – a bath to heal the bond between us. I watched in admiration everything he could do, instead of being over-concerned about him. He also let me comfort him more. Where he used to turn his head away from me when I picked him up, I've found, since the 'rebirth' and the bath ritual, that he increasingly looks for my attention, as if asking me to comfort him.

The other extraordinary result of the coaching sessions is that Tony is not the only man with whom I have a different bond: after the 'rebirth' I spoke to my sperm donor and told him about my ideal birth and that he was present – to my own astonishment. In turn, he told me that he actually would have liked to have been present at the birth, but didn't dare suggest it because this would have been unthinkable for me while I was pregnant. He said he had found me to be unreachable since Tony's birth. He told me he had been very upset when he found out about my depression and that Tony had had to be at the crèche full-time, because he would have liked to play a more active role in Tony's life. He hadn't wanted to impose, however, because we had agreed beforehand that he would keep his distance until Tony asked about him himself. Since that talk, he has slowly taken on a sort of fatherly role and that has been good for all three of us. Tony even spends one day with him every weekend. I use that day to recharge my batteries. When I look back at the dark period, I realise it has brought me so much good. I have become my old sensitive self again, the way I was before I lost my father. People tell me motherhood has softened me. While it undoubtedly plays a role, it's the 'daring to feel again' that has ultimately brought me back to myself." (Lena, 39 years old)

Exercise: Bath-bonding ritual

After the FHER session, clients are advised, when they're ready, to have a healing bath together with their baby and thus to repair the bond between mother (or father) and child. This idea of a healing and wholesome bath for mother and baby was first described by Swiss midwife Brigitte Meissner. In my practice I've also found that it gives exceptional results.

Of course, you can carry out this bath-bonding ritual by yourself. Wait until the moment feels "good". Don't wait until the "perfect" moment because there's no such thing as a perfect moment. A good moment is one when you're relaxed and when you won't be disturbed by other children or by the phone. You can place your baby calmly on your chest. If your child is already older, he can play quietly while you sit together in the bath. You tell your child what it was like when you found out you were pregnant, how stirring it was and which emotions you had during the pregnancy and birth. You don't need to go into the disturbing details of the birth, it's sufficient to say you found it stressful or hard. It doesn't matter if you become emotional or cry, as long as you explain to your child why you're crying. Children aren't usually startled by emotion. It helps to explain to them – even to babies – why you're crying or why you're sad, afraid, or angry, and the fact that it hasn't anything to do with them personally, but with your experience of their birth. You really don't need to tell a long story, your child knows, without too many words, what you're trying to tell him. After you've told your birth story you make a movement of pushing your baby off your chest and into the water and then immediately, in one fluid movement, you bring him back on to your chest. This symbolises the birthing process. You welcome your baby to the world and tell him how happy you are that he's in your life. This doesn't need to last very long either. Just one shared moment is enough and can have a positive and healing effect on your relationship with your child.

It's extra special if your partner can then be ready with a warm towel to wrap you in, and if you can then all three lie on your bed together and share how happy you are with one another. You can also bring up happy memories of the pregnancy, birth, early days or recent fun experiences you've had together. Sometimes, on the other hand, there's no need to talk, it's sufficient just to hold each other or to have skin-on-skin contact as you did just after the birth. If you don't have a partner, step out of the bath with your child on your arm, dry yourself and your baby, put on a bath robe and then lie in bed together under the covers and tell your child again how happy you are with him. If you don't have a bath, you can do this exercise in the shower.

"I had come so far already with the EMDR and the FHER. I thought the bath-bonding ritual sounded a little too much because I already bathed with my children every week. But my curiosity got the better of me because the EMDR and FHER had had such astonishing results. So I waited for the right moment. When our eldest daughter was staying over with her grandparents, I saw my chance. My husband was sceptical about the whole 'bath affair', but agreed to try, because he was happy that I was doing so well again after a long miserable time. My son sat playing in the bath. I wanted to hold him close and tell him his birth story but he resisted. So I let him play instead and started telling him. I became emotional – and he put his toy boats down and came to me without saying anything. I kept talking, and when I came to the moment when he came out of my tummy and then lay on my chest, I pushed him off me and then pulled him back on to me. He looked at me as if to say: *'Was that so hard to say, Mummy? I knew that all along.'* My husband wrapped us up in a warm towel and we all had a wonderful cuddle in bed. A year and a half after giving birth I experienced an ideal birth moment. Since then, my son is much cuddlier than before and I'm a lot more patient with him."
(Margo, 29 years old)

Kate's

STORY

Ten months after the birth of my second child, I noticed that I was stuck. My thoughts and my feeling of failure haunted me. It had been an intense delivery but that hadn't bothered me at first. I was so proud of myself and so happy with our son. It was only afterwards that I began to feel unhappy.

I'm in labour, lying in an uncomfortable position, flat on my back like a banana with my long legs in stirrups. The midwife on duty stands (both literally and figuratively) opposite me. During the pushing stage I feel as though I have to push upwards, against the force of gravity, and the baby doesn't get past my pubic bone. I keep saying that I'm not lying comfortably and that the position is stopping me from pushing effectively. I want to sit up, but the midwife says she wouldn't be able to get to the baby then. She urges me to "give it everything I've got and push through the pain". I was already doing that, and no matter what I try, the baby doesn't budge. After half an hour of pushing, the midwife hands my delivery over to the gynaecologist. She leaves the room for 15 minutes to discuss it and in that time I'm afraid my baby is getting smothered and will run out of oxygen.

The gynaecologist comes in and stands next to me while I push. This makes it seem like we're doing it together and it gives me confidence. I'm given a drip to make the contractions stronger. I'm exhausted and ask my husband for grape sugar tablets. I swallowed three at once. After ten minutes I feel the contractions getting stronger. The gynaecologist guides me with her fingers so that I push in the right direction. She asks me to hold my legs myself and to make as much room as possible in my pelvis for the baby. Three contractions later I can pull my baby out myself. A truly magic moment! The gynaecologist says with a smile: *"that grape sugar really helped you!"* I'm so happy to have a healthy child lying on my chest.

In the week following the birth, my view of the delivery changes and is negatively influenced by the midwives who come to do the postpartum checks. All three of them say something along the lines of *"What a shame that you weren't able to birth your second child by yourself"*, *"A pity you couldn't give birth without extra stimulation"* and the most painful: *"You didn't produce good enough contractions to push with."* I started brooding. Was my positive image of the birth so unfounded? Had I failed? A couple of weeks later, I met a midwife at school who had been on holiday when I gave birth (which is why I had the duty-midwife). When she also used the word "pity" when talking about my delivery, I know for sure that I messed up the birth. I start brooding more and more. We're not planning to have more children, so I won't get another chance to do this birth over. I saw myself as a kind of Earth Mother, made for such an intrinsically maternal event as childbirth. Being a mother to our two children is the best thing that ever happened to me – but I still felt like I had failed at the second birth.

During the coaching sessions it became clear to me what was "mine" (the moment of happiness when I pulled my son out myself, and what was "the midwife's" (the disappointment of having to hand over the birth of a second child to the gynaecologist). These were two separate stories. The midwives shouldn't have shared their side of the story with me without my asking for it, and I shouldn't have let my positive experience be tainted by their opinion.

I was seeing a coach to process my birth experience. She suggested I try EMDR – and I'm so glad that I did! All the emotions that I had been through during the birth came up, one by one: the helplessness, frustration, anger, but also that overriding happiness. I felt the loneliness again but also how good it felt when our son was finally born and I could hold him – how blissful I felt at that moment. No-one can take that bliss away from me. At the end of the session, the coach said she saw a change in my posture during the EMDR, from a hunched-up little mouse to a strong and confident woman.

After the EMDR I was extremely tired, as if I had just given birth again. I went straight to bed when I got home, slept for a long time and had a terrible headache when I woke up the next day. I also felt that things were going to be alright, I felt very confident about that. For about a week after the EMDR, I was moody – I'm glad I had been warned in advance that this could happen.

Just before his first birthday, my son and I had a bath together and I told him how happy I was with him, how strong we were bonded together, how he had been in my tummy and how he was born. I told him how we got through the birth together and how much he was and is a part of my life. After that, it was done, and it was good. My transformation from a nice, polite little mouse to a confident woman is still very evident. The only thing I was "guilty" about with hindsight was being too polite, too nice. Nowadays, when I feel that I'm getting angry, I express it. This gives me space and air. I'm now confident about myself, I say what I mean. I set my boundaries clearly and uphold them. Others can agree with me or not, I have my own opinions and I do what feels right for myself and my family. I am an Earth Mother!

Anne-marie's

My third daughter, Julie, was born unbelievably quickly. Everyone said how lucky I was, but I felt completely besieged by the delivery. Our eldest child was born in hospital after almost 48 hours of labour. The second took almost 24 hours, so I didn't think of myself as a fast "birther". I had planned to give birth in hospital again but this time it didn't go according to plan. At exactly 37 weeks my waters broke. Straight away I had back-to-back contractions. I couldn't stand up anymore, couldn't walk and rolled around on the bed in agony. My husband calmly got our older children's things together to take them to the neighbours' house. He didn't seem to be in any hurry at all. To make things worse, our car was in the garage that day for a maintenance check. I screamed for him to call a taxi and that we had to get to the hospital right away, but he decided to call the midwife first. I resented him so much for that, that he didn't listen to me, didn't take seriously what I was feeling, while I was the one giving birth, not him. I crawled around the bed in blind panic, growling like a dog. The midwife arrived and Julie was born about ten minutes later. The whole thing had lasted less than an hour. I didn't need stitches and had hardly lost any blood. The midwife complimented me on a perfect home birth, but I couldn't comprehend any of it. Before I knew it, I was in the shower, the bed had been cleaned, the dirty bedding was in the wash and my husband, in his enthusiasm, had already collected our daughters from the neighbours. Suddenly my parents and parents-in-law were on the doorstep and I felt like I couldn't breathe. I couldn't put into words how I felt. Luckily they all went away after a while. I looked at my newborn daughter and felt nothing. I didn't recognise her, whereas with my first two children, I had immediately felt they were "mine". A few days later I tried to explain my feelings to the midwife. She told me it was completely normal and that I just needed to get used to the baby, and to recover from what she called my lightning-speed delivery. I said it felt like I had been hit by lightning and laughed at my play-on-words. The midwife laughed along and then the moment passed.

With my first two children the breastfeeding had gone well, but this time it wasn't working. Julie was a very impatient drinker; she kept choking on her milk and then bringing it all up again. I became increasingly irritated and decided to stop breastfeeding. This didn't bother me even though I had breastfed the first two for almost a year. I handed the care of the newborn over to the trainee nurse, who was learning a lot in our busy home. It didn't strike me that this was just an excuse not to have to look after my daughter – and no-one else noticed, apparently. I did what I had to do, said what I had to say and nobody was aware of how empty I felt inside.

Six weeks later I went to the midwife for the postnatal meeting. She gave me a questionnaire about my psychological wellbeing and I saw that the results startled her. She referred me to a coach. *"I feel quite despondent mentally,"* I confided. The coach asked to what extent my sense of despondency had to do with my mother. I burst into tears. It sounds strange, but I actually felt my body react when she said those words. An intense *"Noooo!"*, together with a *"Stay away from that, stay AWAY!"*, while at the same time, a feeling that this was where the answer lay, buried very deep for years. My mother was admitted to a psychiatric hospital with postnatal depression after I – her third daughter – was born. My parents finally got divorced when I was six, and two years after that my mother was killed in a car accident. My sisters and I were brought up by our father, who left our upbringing in the hands of au-pairs. Every year until I was 14, we had a different au-pair, from a different country, with different habits.

Now I had three daughters of my own, I felt empty and was depressed according to the test. I was terrified that history would repeat itself and that I would also have to go to a psychiatric facility. During the coaching sessions I grieved for my mother, for the carefree childhood that I missed out on, and for my irrational feeling of guilt because my mother got sick when I was born. It was an arduous journey but it felt good to clear away the rubble of my youth at last. My mother's unhappy life had frightened me for a long time. My father had painted a picture that motherhood could only be laborious. I did everything in my power not to follow my mother's example and to prove my father wrong in his view of motherhood. I wanted to control everything, in my private life as well as at work. This demanded a tonne of energy. There was no room for spontaneity in my life. I planned everything and was thrown if things didn't go according to my plan. In contrast, my husband was very flexible and easy-going. He let me do all the planning, and just went along with it.

The unplanned, early and quick birth was the last straw that broke my control-donkey's back. I couldn't keep up appearances any longer. It was very hard to move the "controller", who had been in charge of my life since my mother's death, to the back seat. Once I had managed that, however, I found room for a more flexible and spontaneous me. What a relief, both for myself and for those around me!

I processed the birth with the help of EMDR. During the session there was a lot of sadness, I felt incredibly scared, lonely and vulnerable. With hindsight, these were all feelings that I pushed away in my day-to-day life. Me… vulnerable? Afraid? Lonely? Of course not. Everything in my life is always perfectly under control!

It took a week before I felt calm inside. During that week I contacted my coach a couple of times to ask if what I felt was normal: completely exhausted, as if I'd been run over by a truck; empty, but not in a frightening way like during the birth, more like "cleared-up empty". Each time she reassured me. And she was right. Slowly the smoke began to clear. I began to see colours again; everything had looked grey for a long time. My youngest daughter started trying to make contact with me, whereas before I felt that she didn't want anything to do with me and reserved her smiles for her father and sisters. I am liberated from my past at long last. I don't need to compare anymore, just to observe: what is happening concretely and how do I react to it? I have complete freedom of choice and this makes me strong and cheerful. My third daughter liberated me from the wreckage of my painful past. With the powerful events surrounding her birth, she gave a new balance to my life and for that I'm forever grateful to her.

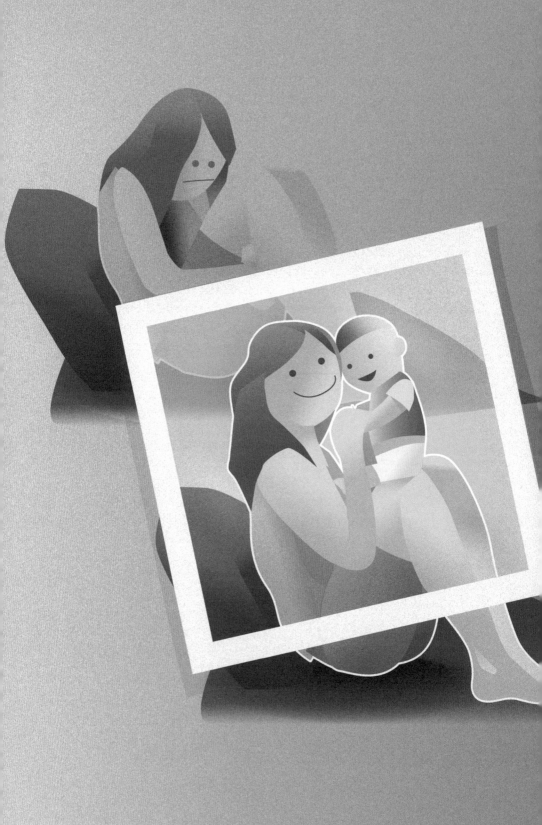

CHAPTER 8

Time for a change

"Men are disturbed not by things, but by the view which they take of them." It isn't the events themselves that make people anxious, sad or stressed but the way people look at these events. The Greek philosopher Epictetus said it almost literally 2,000 years ago. Psychologists call this a "subjective interpretation" of events. An event triggers different thoughts, feelings and behaviour in you than it does in your partner, your best friend or me. By changing the way you think about an event you can also change your behaviour and this gives you new experiences. We all see ourselves, each other and the world through our own lens of experiences.

*"If you keep thinking what you always thought
and keep doing what you always did,
you'll keep seeing what you always saw
and keeping getting what you always got."*

If you look through a different lens and start thinking in a different (helpful, neutral or positive) way, you will behave differently and then your daily life experiences will also be different. Unfortunately we often look at our lives through a negative lens. For example, if you avoid certain situations out of fear, you will never discover that they are not as bad as you had feared. If you feel down or depressed and keep assuming the worst, you're more likely to be defensive or negative. This will make others react defensively, negatively or even with hostility and this in turn can reinforce your negative, unhelpful thoughts and keep you stuck in your negative, unhelpful behaviour. Micha has been feeling low since she became a mother. She can't stand her baby Teddy's crying anymore. On my request she brings Teddy to a coaching session. A couple of minutes into the session, Teddy starts to cry.

Micha reacts as if stung by a wasp. She jumps up, picks Teddy up out of the buggy and starts apologising. She has tears in her eyes. She is upset for Teddy because he's crying, for herself because Teddy is crying, upset for me because Teddy is crying and she's also reacting simultaneously to all the times that Teddy has cried in the past and made her feel hopeless because she couldn't get him to calm down.

She feels miserable and thinks all sorts of negative thoughts at the same time: here we go again; he's going to keep crying through the entire session, I never manage to make him stop anyway; the whole session is ruined, I may as well leave now; what will Diana think of me, she can see now what a terrible mother I am; and – the most painful thought to express out loud – horrid child, you spoil everything with your crying.

As an outsider, I have no previous bad experience of Teddy and his crying. Therefore I can watch the same event from a very different perspective and have very different thoughts about it. I see Teddy crying – nothing more, nothing less. I wonder why he's crying – perhaps he's hungry or needs a nappy change – but I don't have any negative thoughts about myself, Teddy or Micha as the baby's mother.

If we set out the event on paper and compare Micha's and my thoughts and feelings, it looks like this:

1. **The event:**
A few minutes into the coaching session, Teddy begins to cry.

2. **The thoughts:**
Micha:
- here we go again
- he's going to keep crying through the entire session, I never manage to calm him down anyway
- the whole session is ruined, I may as well leave now
- what will Diana think of me, she can see now what a terrible mother I am

- horrid child, you spoil everything with your crying

Diana:
- ah, Teddy is crying
- perhaps he's hungry or needs a nappy change
- I see that Micha jumps up and starts apologising

3. The feelings:

Micha:
- desperation, frustration, anger, sadness
  (tears in her eyes)

Diana:
- curiosity
  (I wonder what's wrong with Teddy)

4. The behaviour:

Micha:
- jumps up, picks Teddy up out of the buggy and tries
  – unsuccessfully – to calm him.

Diana:
- stays calmly in her chair and observes the interaction
  between Micha and Teddy

Teddy:
- feels the tension and worry in his mother and becomes
  even more restless and inconsolable.

Why does Micha behave the way she does and why do I react so differently to the same event? Micha's thoughts and feelings about the event influence her behaviour. Her behaviour in turn creates new negative thoughts and feelings. She could have shared her thoughts with me and asked me what I thought of the situation. Then she would have discovered that my thoughts were much more neutral and positive than hers. Perhaps this would have allowed her to feel less stressed and made her behave differently. Don't assume you know what another person is thinking; check with them that what you think is correct.

It's almost impossible to not think. Thinking is the first thing you do when you wake up and the last thing you do before you fall asleep. Most of the time you're not actually aware of the cascade of thoughts and feelings that are generated in you by an event and you react automatically/subconsciously with a certain behaviour/behavioural pattern: behaviour that has worked for you in the past in a comparable situation.

It's important to identify and place thoughts that are disturbing, negative, forceful ("must"s) and thoughts that hold you back from doing something. This sort of thinking is called black-and-white thinking. Some examples are: *"This will never work"*, *"I've ruined everything"*, *"I'm always unlucky"* and *"No-one ever listens to me"*. Once you have pinpointed your negative thoughts you can learn to bend them into helpful thoughts.

The exercises in this chapter can help you do this. The insights are based on a number of theories of psychology: Rational Emotive Behaviour Therapy (REBT, developed by Albert Ellis), Cognitive Behavioural Therapy (CBT, developed by Aaron T. Beck), *"The Work"* (developed by Byron Katie) and Transactional Analysis (TA, developed by Eric Berne). I complement these theories with practice-based examples and condense them into a completable observation sheet.

Observation sheet

The sheet below can help you to look at the situation/event from a distance and to take a time-out in order to become aware of your thoughts and feelings, before you react. As far as you're concerned, these thoughts are the truth, and you look for and find confirmation of your truth, time after time. That's why you keep reacting in the same way. The sheet will help you identify this kind of unhelpful behaviour. By analysing the situation afterwards you will see which thoughts, feelings or behaviours are helpful or unhelpful in a particular situation.

With (a lot of) practice, you'll be able to become aware of your thoughts and feelings increasingly quickly and eventually to choose the best possible or most appropriate behaviour in response to the event. For most people, this is a life-long process.

1 Event	2 Thoughts	3 Feelings	4 Behaviour (old)	5 Behaviour (new)	6 Successful?
	• Is what you BELIEVE true? • What evidence do you have? • What information is missing?	• Angry • Afraid • Sad • Where in your body do you feel it?		• How would you like to behave?	
....	....	....	....	....	....
....	....	....	....	....	....
....	....	....	....	....	....
....	....	....	....	....	....
....	....	....	....	....	....
....	....	....	....	....	....

Try to be as objective as possible when looking at the initial situation or **event (1)**. Then briefly describe your **thoughts (2)** and **feelings (3)** in response to that event. Write down how you reacted – this is your **old behaviour (4)** – and how you would have liked to have reacted – your **new behaviour (5)**. If your original behaviour is the same as the one you would have liked, you can tick the last box: **successful (6)**. Of course, not every line will begin with an event. In most cases you'll feel something in your body first. Your body gives you signals that it's tense; you might clench your teeth, feel pressure in your chest, a weight in your stomach, pressure in your head etc. The more aware you are of your body's signals, the faster you can work out which feeling the signal corresponds to and what that feeling is trying to tell you. People often jump straight from event to behaviour without being conscious of thoughts and feelings.

The following questions can help you become conscious of them:
- What **happened (1)** just before you started to panic
  or became stressed/anxious/angry/sad?
  Where were you and who was with you?
- Which **thoughts (2)** went through your mind?
- Is what you thought/think true? Are you sure?
  What evidence do you have?
- Did you express your thoughts and check them
  for accuracy with anyone?
- Are you missing any facts that can help you
  to be completely sure?
- What would you like to think?
  What thoughts would be helpful?
- What **feelings (3)** did you have at that moment?
  (for example, shame, guilt, jealousy, irritation)
- Where in your body did you feel the
  tension/stress/panic/fear/anger/sadness?
  (You often automatically place your hand on that part
  of your body if someone asks you this question).
- What did you do?
  What was your **(old) behaviour (4)** like?

- How else could you have reacted/how would you have liked to have reacted? Fill this in under **new behaviour (5)**.

I give my clients this assignment to do every day (!) with at least one example. During each coaching session, we go through the observation sheet. The sheet has many instructions and together we try to identify where the stumbling blocks are and which things we might be able to change. In the beginning it takes a considerable effort for people to put their thoughts and feelings into words (let alone to know how these came about), and to know what they would have wanted their reaction to be. There is a reason that changes in our behaviour take two months on average. It's normal for it to take six to nine months for us to adopt new behaviour. To become aware – and stay aware – of unhelpful/hindering thoughts and to keep transforming these thoughts into helpful, positive ones is a lifelong growth process. It isn't easy to identify irrational or unhelpful thoughts by yourself. After all, to you, your thoughts seem very logical and make perfect sense. A therapist or coach can help you become aware of your thoughts and feelings. You can make an initial appointment with several psychologists or coaches until you find one that you "click" with. If you feel at ease with a therapist who supports you unconditionally and without judgment, you'll be able to make the changes much more quickly.

You might also prefer online therapy, if you find it easier to write down your thoughts, and this is fine, of course. With online therapy you usually have the same therapist each time, but the "click" is less important because most of the communication is done through email.

Here are two examples to illustrate the point:

When you're feeling good emotionally
Event (1):   The baby moves a lot during your pregnancy
Thought (2):   I love all these little kicks!
Feeling (3):   Happiness
Behaviour (4): You rub your belly, talk to your baby, let your
                         partner and loved ones feel the baby moving

When you're not feeling good emotionally
Event (1):   The baby moves a lot during your pregnancy
Thought (2):   It's going to be another hyperactive baby, just
                         like his older brother – I can't handle this!
Feeling (3):   Worry, insecurity
Behaviour (4): You need to be reassured, don't talk to your baby,
                         don't encourage others to make contact with the
                         baby.

When you're feeling good emotionally
Event (1):   The baby cries
Thought (2):   She's hungry/needs to be changed/I know what
                         she needs/I'm a good (enough) mother!
Feeling (3):   Competent, able to calm your baby
Behaviour (4): You meet your baby's needs, the baby stops crying

When you're not feeling good emotionally
Event (1):   The baby cries
Thought (2):   She's doing this to annoy me/I have no idea
                         what's happening/I'm a bad mother
Feeling (3):   Anger, sadness
Behaviour (4): You reject your baby, your baby feels the
                         rejection, her need (clean nappy, food, comfort,
                         burp) is not met, she cries inconsolably.
Result: Instead of comforting your baby, you, as a parent,
unconsciously and involuntarily contribute to your baby's stress.
In turn, your baby will cry more loudly and this increases your
level of stress.

"There used to be an advertisement with grandparents trying to out-do each other by buying their grandchild the biggest, most expensive teddy bear. That's how it was in my family just after I gave birth. Both my mother and my mother-in-law are, to put it mildly, enthusiastically present. Polly was the first grandchild on both sides of the family and they didn't let us forget it. They both had keys to our house and came and went as they pleased. If one did the shopping and cooked a meal, and I accidentally mentioned to the other how well we had eaten, the other would be over the very next day, preparing a three-course meal for us. It was very kind but it was driving me mad.

My coach gave me the questionnaire to fill in. She noticed that almost all the situations involved frustrations about my mother or mother-in-law, or arguments between my husband and me about my mother or mother-in-law. The questionnaire helped me see that too – there must have been six examples in just two weeks. I really needed to learn exactly what I was feeling; in the beginning I kept saying: *"I think that I feel..."*. I found it challenging – and annoying – to fill in the questionnaire. I took out my annoyance on my husband at first, leading to many more examples to fill in! My mother and mother-in-law kept taking Polly out of her cot, at the smallest sound she made in her sleep, supposedly because she was waking up. But I knew they just did that because they wanted to see her awake and to be able to cuddle and purr over her. My coach jokingly called that *"too much love"* and that's exactly what it was. I found myself constantly clenching my teeth and fists, but wasn't able to say anything because I knew how hurt they would be: they meant well. At first I couldn't even imagine how I might behave differently. Usually I would escape to the bedroom with the excuse that I had to breastfeed Polly and she was too easily distracted from her feed.

When I finally opened my mouth, my words were so full of venom, that I made both my mother and my mother-in-law cry. I learned that my body knew before I did that I was irritated. Then I would clench my fists or my teeth. By focusing on what was happening in my body (feeling, 3), I not only became aware of what I was feeling, but I could trace my feelings back to what had happened just before, whatever had irritated me so much. I would sneak a peek at my four-part communication process notes (see Chapter 5) and practise to myself

on the toilet. I felt the irritation, now I had to put into words what I saw or heard, identify my mother(-in-law)'s intention/meaning, understand what this did to me – which feelings it triggered in me – and, the hardest for me, express what I needed at that moment. Often, I found that my boundaries had been crossed long before. I had let it happen, the tension built up, negative thoughts and feelings flowed and then I exploded. To my well-intentioned mother and mother-in-law, this explosion came out of nowhere. Just asking that the radio be turned off in my own house because I wanted to rest my ears, or saying that I wanted to have a day alone with my husband and baby, they seem so simple, but they were real achievements for me. Gradually, I was able to put more ticks in the 'successful' (6) column. Polly grew thanks to my breast milk, and I grew thanks to the coaching."
(Stephanie, 23 years old)

From drama triangle to empowerment dynamic

The drama triangle is one of the most well-known models in Transactional Analysis (TA). If there's friction in a relationship – in any relationship, it can be with your partner, colleague, boss, friend or mother(-in-law) – it can usually be illustrated by a drama triangle. There are three players in a drama triangle: a Persecutor, Rescuer and Victim. You don't always have the same role; in fact, you usually jump from one role to another.
In the example above, there is a drama triangle. Stephanie's mother and mother-in-law are keen to help. Except that they don't help, they rescue, and this makes Stephanie feel like a Victim. Since she doesn't like this role, she becomes irritated and lashes out at the Rescuers (the mothers). Stephanie moves from Victim to Persecutor. The Rescuers feel offended, because they had meant well! Stephanie's verbal attack makes them swap their Rescuer role for a Victim role. And so it goes once you've landed in a drama triangle with someone: you run after one another, each time occupying a different corner and playing a different role, without even realising it.

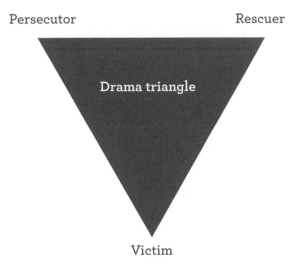

In general, the drama stems from conflict, rage, disappointment and a sense of not being heard, seen or taken seriously.

There are three roles: the Persecutor, Rescuer and Victim.

- The **Persecutor** waves a reproving finger, uses a loud voice and hostile words to say what's not right (usually things he thinks he can do better) and why another person – the Victim – is wrong and deserves to be punished. The Persecutor thinks he's right and can go very far to be proven right. If necessary he will pull other people into the drama triangle. The basic position of the Persecutor is: "I'm okay, you're not okay." Sometimes Persecutors shout loudly in order to hide their own insecurity (or weaknesses).

- The **Rescuer** is only concerned with helping, rescuing, pleasing etc. He makes himself irreplaceable and is convinced that if he's not around to rescue, everything will go wrong. Rescuers answer questions that haven't yet been asked, see solutions where others haven't yet signalled a problem and are always involved in organising things and "just helping out": "Oh, let me do that, it's really no problem." Rescuers like to be trusted and thrive on gratitude for and dependence on their help. Because of this they're, like the Persecutor, not on an equal standing with the person who fulfils the Victim role. Rescuers need Victims in order to feel needed. If Rescuers feel they are dismissed or undervalued, they fall into the role of Victim or Persecutor. Like the Persecutor, the basic position of the Rescuer is: "I'm okay, you're not okay" (because you're attacking me or I need to rescue you, therefore I'm "better" than you).

- The **Victim** is blameless. He is in this position, completely through the fault of others (usually the Persecutor), or of circumstances, like a baby bird that's fallen out of the nest, and he needs a Rescuer to get him out of his distressing position. "I couldn't help it", "It's not my fault", "here we go again, I'm so unlucky" are typically expressed by Victims. If the Rescuer stops rescuing, the Victim feels he's been abandoned. He might then choose to take on the Persecutor role, which pushes the Rescuer into a Victim's role. The original Victim will be looking for a new Rescuer in the meantime. The Victim finds he's not okay, and neither is the Persecutor. The Rescuer is okay as long as the Victim is willing to be rescued, but if the Victim is rescued against his will, the Rescuer is no longer okay. In this case, from the point of view of the Victim, no-one is okay and the world is generally frightening or hard to grasp and therefore also not okay.

In the workshops and training sessions I let the participants think of examples of themselves in all three roles, because we're all in drama triangles and keep moving from one role to another. We see other people's lives through our own lens, which is coloured by our own experiences, and we make assumptions about what other people are thinking, intend or should do. Many mothers recognise themselves at first in the Rescuer role, in relation to their children as well as to their partner. The interesting thing is that children don't want to be Victims at all – they're always striving to do things by themselves. Children are mini-people who, with some help and coaching, can look after themselves perfectly well at their own level of development. Your partner usually doesn't want to be rescued either. He is (usually) a man, and likes to do things his way and in his time. Give him a chance and stay out of the drama triangle.

Finally, the role of Persecutor is not unknown to most parents, especially if they have toddlers or teenagers. You hear yourself complaining and losing control and you know that it doesn't help, but you feel trapped in the drama triangle.

> **Do you have a P-Personality?**
> Are you a Perfectionist?
> Do you try to Perform Perfectly, dutifully make Precious Priority lists and tick them off?
> Do you spend a lot of time Pampering and Pleasing others?
> Do you often take Problems Personally?
> Do you Push yourself to the limit?
> Do you brood every day about what others think of you or about what you could/should have done better?
> Do you tend to Panic when things don't go according to Plan?
> And all this because you think that you need to Perfect your imPerfect Personality, because you wouldn't otherwise be worthy?
> Please stoP!
> Breathe out, let it go and relax.
> Perfection doesn't exist.
> Good is really good enough.
> You really are good enough, Precisely as you are now,
> on your own Path of life!

"I found myself home with a burnout when my youngest son was just a year old. In the first session, the coach asked if I could see myself in this description of a P-Personality.

I burst into tears. Other than the last four lines, the words applied 'perfectly' to me. As a child of divorced parents I had learned to try to keep the peace whenever I could. My parents' wishes took precedence over my own when I had my baby. My father didn't want to come to visit if his new, young girlfriend wasn't welcome. I really didn't want her to waltz in, all fresh and young while I felt so old and tired after my gruelling birth, but I didn't want to offend my father and so put his wishes above my own. My mother didn't want to attend the birth celebration if my father was going to be there with his new girlfriend, so in the end I only invited my friends. I took my baby to the office where there was a disastrous mini celebration. When I arrived, everyone was 'just finishing something off'. A colleague had warned me that the atmosphere was very tense because of the company restructuring. During my maternity leave, five colleagues had left. The new colleagues introduced themselves politely, congratulated me, looked in the pram politely, and then went back to working at their computers with their backs to the party. I felt like a stranger in my own office. When I went back to work, everyone around me was complaining. I had taken parental leave but the amount of work had not been adjusted so I was doing four days' worth of work in three days. My manager, whom I liked, had left during my maternity leave and been replaced by an interim-manager whom I hardly ever saw smile in the whole six months I worked with her. I wanted to be useful but got lost in priority lists, which made me less and less productive. I began to brood, slept badly and went off track.

In the coaching sessions I was introduced to the drama triangle. I immediately recognised my situation with my parents and my role at work. In both cases I tried to rescue what was left to salvage. My new manager was the Persecutor and when my rescuing attempts failed, I was the Victim. My father presented himself sometimes as the Victim and sometimes as the Persecutor, and I swung between Rescuer and Victim. The combination of failed rescue attempts and being a Victim had led to my burnout. I learned to separate what concerned me and what was the concern of others (my father, manager or company). I concentrated on the things I could influence. Not everything was my problem or my responsibility. Luckily, I soon got a new manager and working at the office became restful again. I have also become much more assertive towards my parents. It's not my problem that they can't be in the same room at the same time. I decide when I host a party and they can decide whether they come or not."
(Yvette, 40 years old)

Assignment:

Think of examples of your own drama triangles. These can be in your family, at work or other relationships such as with your parents (-in-law) or acquaintances.

Persecutor's role:
- In relation to:

  ....
- What sentences do you hear yourself say when you're in the Persecutor's role?

  ....
- In which role is the other person at that moment?

  ....

Rescuer's role:
- In relation to:

  ....
- What sentences do you hear yourself say when you're in the Rescuer's role?

  ....
- In which role is the other person at that moment?

  ....

Victim's role:
- In relation to:

  ....
- What sentences do you hear yourself say when you're in the Victim's role?

  ....
- In which role is the other person at that moment?

  ....

In the example above, Yvette clearly explains how she moved between the Rescuer and Victim while her father and manager were mostly in the Persecutor role. There are only losers in a drama triangle relationship. A round of punches leaves everyone feeling bad. Yvette managed to step out of the drama triangle with the help of the coaching sessions. This forced her manager and her parents to step out of it too and they entered instead into the opposite triangle. Fortunately this exists too: the empowerment dynamic. In this triangle, all the roles have equal standing.

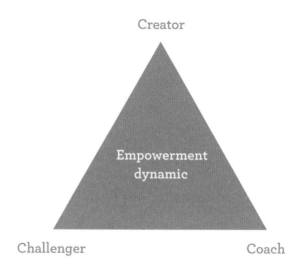

The Persecutor becomes a Challenger who offers clarity, sets out his boundaries and guards them, but also accepts and respects the boundaries of others. Rather than using accusing "you-sentences", express what you see/think and what you need using I-sentences".

The Rescuer presents himself as a Coach. He helps others – only when asked – to get the best out of themselves. He is caring rather than overprotective, involved rather than interfering, he empathises instead of taking on part of the suffering. He does what is asked of him and what he has promised, nothing more and nothing less. He assumes that others can look after themselves. He coaches because he likes to, not because he craves gratitude or recognition.

In the empowerment triangle, the Victim turns into a Creator: he questions what is possible and what isn't. What do I need or have to learn in order to manage on my own? He can ask for help, but from a position of equality, not one of inferiority. Everything he tries or learns increases his self-confidence.

Assignment:
How can you get from your role in the drama triangle to the corresponding role in the growth triangle?

Challenging role:
- In relation to:
....
- What sentences do you hear yourself say when you're in the Persecutor's role?
....
- In which role is the other person at that moment?
....

Coaching role:
- In relation to:
....
- What sentences do you hear yourself say when you're in the Rescuer's role?
....
- In which role is the other person at that moment?
....

Creating role:
- In relation to:
....
- What sentences do you hear yourself say when you're in the Victim's role?
....
- In which role is the other person at that moment?
....

In my practice I often see that women react in a submissive manner: while their words seem neutral and friendly they have a nasty undertone. *"Sure, I'll do that. No problem"*, said in a slightly annoyed tone, through clenched teeth and with a frown, while they grumble silently. Or their words say *"yes"* and their actions say *"no"*. When you learn new behaviour, you often go overboard a bit at first. From being submissive you might well plunge straight into aggressive behaviour, with people around you getting criticism thrown in their faces. In the end you should be able to find the middle position, neither submissive nor aggressive, but assertive. You say what you mean, do what you promise, and express your needs. Nothing more, nothing less. You don't need to be unpleasant about it; on the contrary, you can be very friendly while being very clear.

Isis's

STORY

My baby daughter, Faith, lay on my belly. I was completely
happy, content and proud. The birth had been intense, tough
and all-encompassing and now she was here. What an amazing
feeling; it was the crowning of our love. My husband and I
admired our daughter, we kissed and suddenly I laughed,
cried and coughed with happiness at the same time. Then I
felt something leaking – leaking heavily. We were alone in the
room. I asked my husband to look under the blanket and saw
him recoil from shock. He told me afterwards that he had seen
the blood stain already coming through the blanket. He ran
out to call for help and soon the room was full of people. I felt
dizzy and asked my husband to take Faith from me. The sounds
in the room were coming from further and further away, as if
I were under water. The medicines they gave me to make my
uterus contract and stop the bleeding had no effect. A nurse
pushed hard down on my belly to squeeze the uterus but that
didn't help either. Before I knew what was happening I was
being wheeled into the operating room. I remember very little
of it. I didn't really care either. It was okay, however crazy that
might sound.

They operated on me for almost three hours. I woke up in
Intensive Care and remembered almost nothing of the whole
delivery. Someone had stuck a picture of my daughter to the
shelf next to me, but I had no concept of time or place, let
alone the fact that I had given birth. My physical recovery
went quite quickly after two blood transfusions, but mentally
I was completely off track. I looked at Faith and at my
husband and thought: what happened? The hospital offered
me psychological support, which I found to be helpful. I had

some EMDR to process the birth, but that didn't take away the strange and unreal feeling I had had since the birth. Strange as it might sound, I didn't have negative feelings about the birth. It was more like a fog. Conversations with the health professionals who had been involved helped me put together the puzzle pieces. I was very happy with the photos my husband had taken during and after the birth – I was in them, so I must have given birth. I should be happy, and I was, but it felt unreal.

I was given extra sick leave from work. Faith was doing well, even though the breastfeeding had never really taken off. The midwife had told me: *"What you don't have, you can't give away. You first need to get your own strength back."* That sounded logical and gave me something to hold on to. And yes, life goes on.

I went back to work – which I was happy about. Except that I had slept badly since the birth and was therefore so tired... so indescribably tired. I made it through the days on willpower and I sometimes felt like a zombie. I could hardly concentrate and had headaches almost every day. I was incontinent since the birth but had heard from friends that that wasn't so uncommon. I also felt like my whole hormone factory had gone wild. I had hot flushes, followed by heart palpitations, felt rushed and then was as nauseous and lethargic as in my first months of pregnancy. I also started losing my hair. The GP couldn't find a reason for my symptoms.

After about ten months of worrying about my health, it was only getting worse. I found a coach through my work doctor. The test she gave me showed me to have depression and anxiety. From the questionnaire I had filled in before the first meeting, she suspected that there may have been a physical cause that was making me feel so bad. She asked what I myself thought was the matter with me. I said it felt like there had been a short-circuit in my body during the birth and that

I had been rewired incorrectly since then. She said she could understand that I had had a psychological knock from all the confusing physical symptoms, that the cause of my problems might be physical and that the feelings of depression and anxiety might be a consequence of it. She also asked if I still trusted my body. The questions made me very emotional. Since the birth I really didn't trust my body anymore. I had been so proud that such a beautiful baby had been able to grow in my body and that I was able to bring her into the world, but after that my body had let me down and I had nearly bled to death. I nearly died! At the age of 28! After having my first child! Since then, I was indeed constantly checking my body. What was I feeling and what was causing all these symptoms? Was it really all psychological as the GP had implied? I had never had psychological problems before. I was healthy and had continued to exercise right up until my maternity leave.

The coach sent me back to the GP, who referred me to an internist. The assistant phoned me that same day: my thyroid was overactive, I had deficiencies in vitamins D and B and the hormone levels in my blood were abnormal. It turned out that after the birth they had only checked my iron and infection levels and those had been okay. My thyroid wasn't enlarged – the GP had felt for that already. Apparently you can still have an overactive thyroid, even if it's not visibly enlarged. I cried with relief: I wasn't mad or depressed, and my hormones were all messed up – just as I had suspected. I had guessed correctly. I was referred to an internist, a gynaecologist and a pelvic floor specialist for the incontinence. I swallowed a load of pills every day: vitamin B complex, vitamin D and I went back on to the birth control pill for a while to get my hormones back on track. I also used a daylight therapy lamp every day for a couple of weeks and went for a strenuous walk with Faith every day. The birth control pill helped enormously with my hormonal imbalance. The pelvic floor therapy almost fixed my incontinence – I only had a problem if I sneezed or coughed. The thyroid was the hardest to treat. First it was overactive and the medication made it underactive. I had to take time off work because I felt as sick as a dog. Eventually they found I had a thyroid infection. This apparently happens to one in ten women after childbirth. I had never heard of it and neither had my friends. The focus was now on my physical recovery. The birth itself hadn't been disastrous but with hindsight, the first year of Faith's life was terribly heavy to bear. She was a year old and I still wasn't myself. By filling in the drama triangle questionnaire I realised how I had put myself into the Victim role for the past year. It was terrible that this had all happened to me, but I was gaining nothing by dwelling on it. It had been a rough year but there was nothing I could change about it now. I cried: *"I don't want this, I don't want this"*, while my coach very calmly repeated: *"But it is the way it is."* Painful but true. I had gathered a whole army of Rescuers around me. In the following session we did an exercise to symbolically close this period. I literally left the misery behind me and taught myself to look forward again with a positive mindset. Whenever I felt myself falling back into the Victim role, I played the song "Let it go" on full volume and sang along at the top of my voice. I consciously stepped out of the drama triangle, took a step to the side and then a step forward, into the empowerment triangle. I taught myself to see myself as a Creator. What was I able to do? What made me happy again? Which aspects of my day had gone well? I wrote these down in my notebook. I also filled in the questionnaire at least once a day and we discussed the situations in the following coaching session. I noticed in the questionnaire that I got irritated at everything and everyone. By writing it down I was able to see the pattern. When something happened that irritated me, I didn't say anything until I exploded. Increasingly I managed to react differently and more assertively. It was good to see progress also in this area – not every day, but every month.

Only sleep remained a problem. I woke up a few times every night and lay staring at the ceiling from 4am or 5am, getting exasperated with my husband's snoring. I had started sleeping in the spare room but that didn't help. I was fed up with it all, fed up with being sick, tired and pitiful. My insomnia was the focus of one of the coaching sessions. The coach said that it seemed as if I was already frustrated when I woke up in the night and looked at the clock, and that my adrenaline level made it biologically impossible for me to fall asleep again. So, my frustration about not sleeping was stopping me from sleeping! I did an exercise to feel my frustration and to embrace it, instead of fighting against it. After that I symbolically swept the frustration out of the window and replaced it in my head with acceptance. If I woke up early in the morning I thought: "Okay, I'm ready for the day", instead of thinking that I was frustrated. If I woke up too early, I did a relaxation exercise or read a book. If that didn't help I would get up, do some laundry, fold and iron while listening to music on my headphones. At least this way I was getting things done around the house. The first time that I slept through the night and was woken up at 6am by Faith's crying was a day to celebrate!

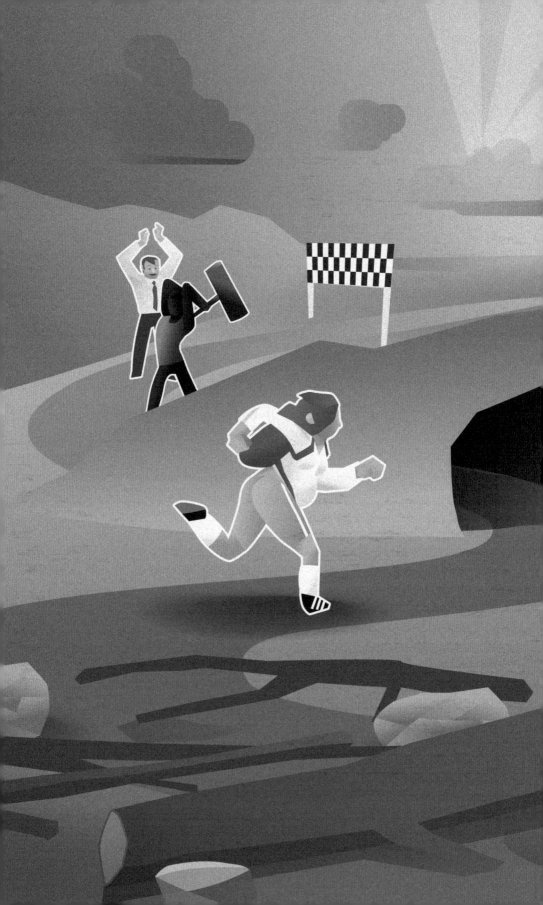

CHAPTER 9

Preparing for the next birth

Looking back and ahead

When you've had a distressing birth experience, it's extra important to prepare yourself for the next time you need to give birth. A pleasant birth experience can partially "repair" a previous one, hopefully letting you remember both of them with a good feeling. Unfortunately, no amount of preparation, birth plan or pregnancy course can guarantee you a good experience.

Answer these questions with your previous delivery in mind:
- What went well during your last birth?
- What would you definitely want to do again?
- What would you like to do differently or avoid this time around?
- What was the worst moment of your last delivery?
- What was it about that moment that was so bad for you?
- What could you yourself do or think differently to avoid having the same bad experience again?
- What could the healthcare professionals do differently?
- Which medical precautions could they take, or could you take together this time?
- Which factors can you influence, and which factors are beyond your influence?

I often see that clients who are preparing for childbirth worry about aspects they have little or no influence over. This is a waste of energy. You're better off spending your energy on factors that you can change.

From feeling you've failed to just being disappointed

The most important thing you can do is to neutralise or transform the way you think about your previous negative experience. You can use this book or a therapist for this. The goal is to go from feeling you have failed (I didn't perform well, it was my fault) to being disappointed (I was unlucky, the baby was badly positioned, the contractions weren't strong enough, or the circumstances were far from optimal). This makes a world of difference to your experience and the way you judge yourself.

Before you give birth again, take the time to rid yourself of self-blame and leave behind any feelings of shame or guilt you may have with regard to your delivery. In doing this, you avoid putting yourself in an already heightened state of awareness at the start of your next labour. This state causes you to feel more pain and to be less tolerant of that pain and makes you vulnerable to distressing memories of your last birth.

Of course, you can't plan a birth and, as the title of this book says, there's no such thing as perfection in childbirth. If you can put together a rough framework with your doctor or midwife and agree on certain things that would make you feel as comfortable as possible, you'll increase your chances of having a positive birth experience. Your midwife or gynaecologist should be aware of what's important for you. During labour, they can contribute to creating optimal circumstances for you, so that you can relax and focus on the job of birthing your baby. If you have particular wishes that aren't easy to carry out, you can come up with a Plan B (or even Plan C) together with your healthcare provider.

CPE

You can also prepare for the next birth using the CPE method. The C stands for Clarity: what are you going to do or planning to do; when, where, why and with whom? The P stands for Practise, because if you don't practise, it will be almost impossible to reach your goal. The most important letter in this acronym is E, which stands for Enjoy. I always ask my clients, *"What are you most looking forward to?"* In response they automatically formulate their goal in a positive way. "To endure the birth" doesn't sound like something that makes you happy. What was your goal in getting pregnant? It probably wasn't to give birth again, but out of a desire to have a child. By focusing on and looking forward to your goal (holding your baby in your arms), you see beyond the delivery. The delivery then becomes a means to achieve your goal, not the goal in itself.

It can help to put yourself in your baby's position. How do you think he/she would like to be born? With a lot of ceremony and intervention, or as calmly and naturally as possible? In order to visualise your goal more clearly and to help encourage you through the upcoming birth, choose a photo or some other object that symbolises a cherished moment of motherhood for you and that makes you smile. If you decide to use a photo, try to find one with you and your baby on it, and, if possible, also your partner. During labour, hold the picture up, literally and figuratively before your eyes. The more effectively and powerfully it produces the corresponding feeling of happiness, the more the image will motivate you. Focusing on a positive goal helps ease the pain: you feel less pain and can also tolerate it better. This is in contrast with being afraid of the pain or focusing on the pain in each contraction. Fear of pain lowers your pain threshold, i.e. the point at which you start feeling the pain. Fear also lowers pain tolerance – the amount of pain you're prepared to bear.

"I made a list of everything that went wrong (or as my coach says, *"things that could have gone differently"*), the first time. For some items I found a solution together with my partner, and for other things the midwife came up with an alternative. My husband had a very passive role during the first birth and I was disappointed by his lack of support. Afterwards he told me he was afraid that the birth of our eldest child was going to go wrong because it was taking much longer than he had expected. To help him feel calm, he went to sit quietly on a chair by the window and played with his phone. He didn't think he could do anything else to help me anyway. I had felt so let down by him... We took on the second birth much more together, which felt good. My husband first massaged my feet and then my lower back. While I was pushing, he sat behind me and applied counter-pressure on my lower back. This made me feel that I could push much harder. I felt supported by him, both literally and figuratively.

During the first labour I had had very intense but short contractions that didn't dilate my cervix efficiently, so I wasn't able to have a home birth. The intensity of the contractions made me trip on the stairs in our house and then again down on the street. In the hospital I had to lie flat on my back, which I found to be a very uncomfortable as well as unnatural position. During the second labour I walked around for as long as I could, leaning over the stairs, on a stool under the shower and eventually had the baby in our living room on the midwife's birthing stool. Our daughter almost slid out by herself on to the birthing stool. Delivering a baby can also be that easy!" (Doreen, 34 years old)

Oxytocin

Oxytocin is the hormone that not only creates strong contractions, but also fosters bonding with others and rest for yourself. This is why it's also called the cuddle hormone. Under the influence of oxytocin, your heart rate and blood pressure go down, you can enjoy pleasant moments more and you have a higher pain threshold. In contrast, the stress hormone, adrenaline, gives you a feeling of anxiety and of being chased, which lowers your pain threshold. You can see why oxytocin is so important during childbirth. Touch, yoga, meditation, mindfulness, sex, massage and a warm shower or bath help you to relax and increase your oxytocin production. The greater the feeling of relaxation you take into the birth, the greater the chance that your own oxytocin production will generate optimal contractions. A positive cycle is created that benefits both you and your baby. Moreover, oxytocin works ingeniously together with endorphins.

Endorphins, a gift from nature

Endorphins are nature's painkillers. They give you a relaxed, almost sleepy feeling, as if you're in a trance. Happy people appear to have more endorphin receptors, making them feel less pain and able to tolerate more pain. During pregnancy your body automatically makes more endorphins in preparation for the intensity of the last stretch. Extra receptors form in your brain, which bind to endorphins so that you can work more effectively with this hormone. During labour you produce more and more endorphins, which give you a natural high. If you picture your contractions as mountains, the endorphins put the mountains under water: you feel the contraction pain a bit later and the pain also stops earlier, as if you've turned down the volume button on your pain system. The more relaxed you are, the more endorphins are produced. The further your labour progresses, the more endorphins are produced, enabling you to endure the increasing pain.

This doesn't work with induced labour. In that case, synthetic oxytocin is released into your bloodstream through a drip. Your body reacts differently to this than to natural oxytocin, and your endorphin system also works differently. There are many factors that come into play, but it's thought that because of this, there is an increased need for painkillers when labour is artificially induced.

Marathon

When athletes run a marathon, they've been training for months and they plan their race in advance as meticulously as possible. They need to pace themselves and divide their energy over 42 kilometres. At a certain point in the race they enter a kind of rhythm at which point the body's production of endorphins is optimal. This is called a "runner's high". But almost all runners also come up against the "man with the hammer". That's when the muscles burn and cramp up and the mind refuses to take another step. Athletes know that this can – and most probably will – happen, and prepare themselves for that difficult moment. For example, they might ask their partner or coach to stand at the point where they expect it to hit. They get through this most difficult part of the race and gather enough courage and energy to reach the finish line. Now, imagine if the finish line of a marathon is flexible, that the organisers suddenly decide to push it back by a couple of kilometres. The marathon runners would probably find it extremely hard to complete that extra stretch because they hadn't accounted or trained for it.

With childbirth there is no fixed finish line and nobody knows how long the "race" will last. That makes it very hard to plan it perfectly. How should you spread out your energy when you don't know how much energy you're going to need or how long you will be in labour? You have no idea in advance how intense it will be, how much energy you have stored, how much strength you'll need for the last part, if and how your muscles will ache and how you'll deal with the pain. In short: you can't plan your birth in advance in the same way runners can plan a marathon. You can, however, try to have the optimal circumstances in place, maximising the chance that you'll get into a flow and your endorphins will give you a kind of runner's high. The calmer the environment and the circumstances, the more confidence you have in yourself and those around you, the higher the chance you'll find yourself in a positive birthing flow. You can also think beforehand about what you'll do if you come across the "man with the hammer" and find that your muscles are cramping up or your mind cramps up and refuses to continue. Who can be your coach at such a moment? What can he or she say to you, between contractions, to make your confidence grow back, to inspire you to climb up and above yourself?

The role of the partner

As a partner, you aren't pregnant but you are expecting. It's good to think, before the birth, about the expectations that you as partners have of each other with regard to the birth and the pain that goes with it. Ask your partner what he (or she) is looking forward to and what he's afraid about. Ask what role your partner sees for himself and also tell him what role you see for him. You are having a baby together. It isn't easy for your partner to see you suffering pain. Sometimes it can be so painful for a partner to see you in pain that they ask for pain medication for you, whereas in fact they cannot bear the pain. Suffering together doesn't actually help the woman in labour; support and sympathy do. In practice, it works best if bystanders at a birth are as calm as possible. The calmer they are, the less adrenaline they have in their own blood, and the less adrenaline you produce. Agitation creates agitation, and calmness around a labouring woman is also contagious. This is not only the case for you partner, but also the healthcare providers who are present while you're giving birth. The more positivity, trust, calm and pleasure in their job that they radiate, the more positive, confident and relaxed the mother-to-be will feel. The role of the partner during childbirth is often underestimated but can be decisive. This is not just a passive supporting role. Active support can consist of touching, literal support, massage for the back, shoulders, legs, hands and feet, pep talks, breathing exercises, positive encouragement but also protection against the outside world. As a partner you uphold your partner's interests if she can no longer do it herself. You can make sure that healthcare providers respect her wishes (insofar as they are medically possible and appropriate). The better you prepare yourself together with your partner, the better you can help and support her. If you, as partner, are dreading the birth, bring this up during the pregnancy check-ups. If you require more (technical) information about the birth, feel free to ask questions. You can also follow a pregnancy or birth preparation course or a few individual lessons together. As a positive, calm and supportive partner, you radiate confidence towards your wife and the birth process. This is one way in which you can make a difference!

Truth and myths about (labour) pain

Many women think they have to decide beforehand if they want to give birth with or without pain. This is actually untrue. It's normal to experience pain during childbirth, but not to suffer pain. Experiencing pain means you are in control of the pain; suffering pain means the pain is in control of you. The best approach is usually to view the pain with wonderment and curiosity. This is a beautiful open position from which you can have new experiences.

Wonderment contains the word "wonder". If the birth goes smoothly there is hardly a need to intervene. Pain is there for a reason. It warns you that something is happening to your body: that you're sick or injured or that you're going to have a baby. Pain gives you a signal that you need to find a safe place and forces you to think (what is this pain trying to tell me?) and to adjust your behaviour (for example, to change position if you have a backache or to rest a sore leg if you can). Many things we learned to do as children, such as walking or riding a bike, involve falling (and being hurt) and getting up again. If your body feels that you're not listening to its signals (like with head or back pain), it might raise the pain level by a peg. In this way, pain forces you to listen to your body and to find a restful place. To ignore the pain, to push it away or to fight it makes it increase.

The media incorrectly depicts childbirth pain as completely unnecessary and outdated. Pain (during labour) makes your body adjust by increasing the hormone levels (oxytocin and endorphins). These hormones are necessary for your baby to be born. However, if the pain becomes too intense (and makes you suffer excessively), you become stressed. Your body then produces stress hormones, adrenaline and cortisol, which work against the positive birthing hormones, oxytocin and endorphins. A bit of tension or stress is fine: it puts your body in a position to carry out this amazing feat (as with marathon runners). But too much stress slows down the birth process, leaving your muscles aching and cramped and making you exhausted. If this happens, pain relief can be valuable. Therefore, let your doctor or midwife know if you're becoming too stressed, if you're in too much pain, or if you're reaching a point of exhaustion. It's important to know that pain relief doesn't address the emotional side of the pain. The word says it all: pain relief relieves pain, not anxiety or the loss of control. Not all women feel better when they feel less pain. On the contrary, medication that numbs the pain can sometimes make you feel more helpless and anxious. Pain relief also cuts off the natural hormonal stream in your body, which can slow the contractions. On the other hand, pain relief can also mean the difference between a bearable birth experience and a traumatic one. You alone can feel your (contraction) pain, so you alone can say what you need to manage your pain.

Ask yourself the following questions before the birth:
- How sensitive are you to pain? Which experiences of pain have led you to this conclusion about yourself?
- Which feelings/emotions are triggered in you by pain? For example, *"Pain frightens me"* or *"I just don't want to have to have any pain at all"*.
- What experiences of pain have you had in the past?
- What ideas have you got from friends, family and the media about pain during labour?
- How do these (often negative) stories influence your attitude

towards pain during labour?

- How do you think you will deal with the pain?
Remember: a contraction lasts approximately one minute, then you have a break of about three minutes to recover. One and three! Focus on the time between contractions. At the start of labour you have about 12 contractions of one minute per hour and 48 minutes with no contractions in that same hour. In the worst phase, between seven and ten centimetres of dilation, you'll have at most 20 contractions in an hour, leaving twice that time to recover from each contraction-you-never-have-to-feel-again.
- How are you going to reflect your (internal) pain in your (external) behaviour? This can be by moving around, rocking, making sounds, grimacing or growling, hitting a pillow, squeezing your partner's hand or arms. It will work against you if inwardly you're crumbling from the pain but not showing it outwardly because you're ashamed of what others might think.
- On a scale of 1 to 10: how much pain do you think there will be at the birth? And on that same scale from 1 to 10, how much pain do you think you can bear? If, for example, you think the pain will be a 10 and you expect that you can bear a maximum of an 8, it would be smart to take some time during your pregnancy to think about how you can get from the 8 to a 9 or 10. What would you need for that? What are you still missing?

You can prepare for the birth using coaching, mindfulness, hypnobirthing, haptonomy, yoga, birthing together or another kind of birth preparation course. This can happen in groups or private courses together with your partner. What's clear is that the way you deal with pain is determined by your expectations of the pain, your attitude towards it and the different ways you think you might deal with it. It also helps to discuss your expectations with your midwife or gynaecologist. The better prepared you are, the more different ways you have of dealing with contractions, and the more realistic your expectations of the pain are, the better you'll be able to bear the pain.

Moreover, psychological, physiological, cultural and environmental factors also play a role. It helps to discuss with your partner and/or your midwife or gynaecologist which of these factors might play a role in your case. If, for example, you don't get on well with your mother-in-law, her presence during your labour might have a negative impact on your mood, the amount of pain you feel and your ability to bear the pain.

Exercise: simulate contractions with an ice-bath for your hand

You can try this 15-minute exercise together with your partner, and it's good preparation for dealing with pain in the first stage of labour. For one minute – because a contraction lasts about one minute – hold your hand in a basin full of ice-cubes with a bit of water. During labour you'll have a contraction of one minute followed by a two- or three-minute break. Therefore, keep your hand repeatedly in the ice water for one minute, followed by a two- or three-minute break out of the water. Having your hand in iced water somewhat resembles the pain of a contraction. Try out the different breathing techniques you've learned to see what pain-relieving effect they have. Does it help to open or close your eyes? Does it help to smile, to sing, or to growl or curse during that one minute that your hand is in the iced water? Does it help to hum or pant the song "twinkle twinkle little star"? Does it help you to be silent, to close yourself off and to have a restful and inspiring image in front of you? Perhaps it helps to defy that one minute when your hand is in the water or are you able to focus in that minute on a part of your body that isn't in pain (a part other than your hand)? Can you endure the one minute every time by focusing on the three minutes that will follow, the three minutes that your hand can be out of the water and your pain system can be at rest again? It has been proven that a positive focus (such as singing, moving around, humming, visualising and smiling) helps to produce more endorphins, allowing you to tolerate more pain. You'll probably notice that you need all your powers of concentration to deal with the pain, making you less alert to what's going on around you. The focus shifts from the outside to the inside.

The EPI-NO

You can increase your feeling of power or control at the pushing stage (the second stage of labour) by practising with a so-called birth trainer or EPI-NO. The birth trainer consists of an anatomically shaped silicon balloon and a hand-held pump. You insert the balloon into your vagina and gradually blow the balloon up using the pump. This improves the blood circulation in your pelvic floor muscles, you train these muscles for the second (pushing) stage and gently stretch the muscles around your vagina. You then push the inflated balloon out yourself and place it on the card to measure how many centimetres (diameter) you reached. The baby's head has a diameter of about ten centimetres. It can give you a lot of (self-)confidence to know that you can already reach six, seven or eight centimetres with the help of the birth trainer. Scientific studies contradict each other on the evidence of the effectiveness of the EPI-NO. In my practice, I have found that the birth trainer can contribute to a woman's (self-)confidence. Confidence enables you to let go of the need to control, and helps you to surrender to the birth process, thus increasing the chance of a positive birth experience.

Gate control and "pain highways"

According to researchers Melzack and Wall, there are two "gates" in the brain and spinal cord that determine which pain stimuli go through and which don't. In their so-called Gate Control Theory, they suggest that gates in the brain can open and close. And the best part is that you can influence this process psychologically.

The brain works as a sort of post room and decides which pain signals need to be communicated urgently and which can wait. This mostly happens subconsciously, but you can also (re)programme your own post room, whereby you consciously determine the priority and intensity of the pain stimulus. There are "urgent pain fibres" from your skin and finger tips that, for example, make you pull back your hand quickly if you get burnt. The deep pain fibres in the uterus travel through a less urgent "post route". They cause a more intense pain but you are aware of it more gradually. The functioning of the TENS (Transcutaneous Electrical Nerve Stimulation) machine is based on this Gate Control Theory. This machine can help you feel less pain. Harmless electric shocks on the skin stimulate the "fast" pain fibres so that you don't feel the "deep" pain from the uterus so much. You might find that you sometimes instinctively create small pain sensations to distract your pain from bigger pain, for example, at the dentist. While at the dentist, many people push their nails into their fingertips or into their palms in order to distract their thoughts from the pain in their mouth. You can borrow or rent a TENS machine from some midwife practices. You can also buy wide-toothed wooden combs to squeeze during a contraction, which stimulates the urgent pain fibres so that you feel the deeper pain from the uterus less.

The old brain

When you give birth you use your "old" brain (limbic system). In daily life you mainly use "new" parts of the brain (the neocortex). This means that you have to switch from using one part of your brain to another during labour. You close yourself off from the world and turn off your "new" brain. High-level athletes can finish a race even after they have been seriously injured. People getting tattoos or cosmetic surgery are so focused on the result that they don't feel the pain so much. If you're able to focus on your goal (holding your baby) instead of focusing on your fear of being in pain, losing control or having complications, you have a much greater chance of having a positive birth experience. This is because focusing on your goal has the effect of numbing the pain, while focusing on the pain amplifies it. Fear lowers your pain threshold (the point at which you start feeling pain) and pain tolerance (the maximum pain you can bear). Fear focuses on what can go wrong (the thistles) instead of seeing what you can do to help yourself (by concentrating on the roses). The most important thing, however, is to have realistic expectations about the (pain of the) birth. The more your brain is focused on the negative aspects of the pain, the more brain activity shows up on a scan with respect to the organs/tissues related to the pain. This makes you feel more pain. Luckily it also works the other way round: by maintaining control over the pain and how you deal with it, you can say what you need and when. That's how you stay on top of the pain!

Fear of giving birth

The arch-enemy of endorphins is stress. Stress slows the production of endorphins. It's normal to be somewhat nervous or a little afraid of going into labour. Fear is a very useful emotion that warns us about danger so that we don't take too big risks or behave carelessly. Fear also gives us the strength and extra energy to deal with dangerous situations. It triggers our fight-or-flight reaction, enabling us to perform better. Healthy fear and healthy tension help you to climb above yourself, both mentally and physically. Many women experience this during childbirth.

When you're stressed, your adrenal glands produce stress hormones. These cause your heart to beat faster and your blood to circulate more quickly, feeding your muscles extra oxygen and glucose (as fuel) to be able to perform better. During such a performance, you automatically switch over to a sort of tunnel vision. Just like a professional athlete, you can concentrate only on your performance. The outside world becomes insignificant at that moment.

If you place someone who is performing in that way into a brain scanner, you will notice frantic activity in the amygdala (part of the limbic system, where the fight-or-flight reflex is located), while the neocortex (the "new" brain, which you use for rational thought) is much less active. The language centre in your brain (Broca's area) doesn't function optimally either. That's why women often have trouble putting into words exactly what happened during the birth. They literally have "no words for it". Due to the pain, the high state of awareness that your body is in and the considerable feat you're undertaking, you can concentrate your attention only on your contractions. Your digestive system becomes of secondary importance; your body can't give it any attention at that moment. That's the reason many women vomit while in labour.

As mentioned earlier, (too much) fear works against you, as it makes your brain go into fight-flight-freeze mode. The more stress hormones there are, the longer and more painful the birth can be. You can tolerate less, your muscles can take less strain and the contractions aren't as effective... you find yourself in a negative vicious circle. Luckily, there is something you can do about this sort of fear of childbirth: discuss it with your midwife or doctor. She can help you put your worry into perspective and to turn that fear into confidence. You can also make an appointment with a midwife-coach who is specialised in guiding women who are worried about giving birth.

"The first time I gave birth I mainly felt angry, because it was going so differently from what I had been made to expect from the pregnancy yoga course. The yoga teacher had said that many of her clients had a virtually pain-free birth after taking her course. For me it was painful – extremely painful. There was no gradual build-up of the pace and intensity of the contractions, it suddenly exploded soon after my waters were broken: two-minute-long contractions that the midwife called 'camel-back' contractions; lots of contractions, but no dilation. I mainly felt the contractions in my legs and back and apparently these are known for being extremely painful but don't dilate the cervix. I felt cheated and unprepared. At the hospital I was soon given an epidural, which gave me some breathing room but it also slowed down the contractions. I was then put on a drip to stimulate the contractions again but that gave me fever and nausea and the baby's heart rate was erratic. In the end I needed a pump, which got my baby out, with a big pointy head.

After the delivery I remained angry. At work too I was very irritable. My colleagues asked me, during a management meeting, if I would be interested in following an anger management course as my team had complained about my short fuse and fierce outbursts. Before having a baby I was known as one of the most emotionally stable managers in the office. During the coaching sessions I learned that I often acted 'nice' while on the inside I was actually very angry or annoyed. When my parents got divorced, I taught myself to 'be nice' and to bury my anger. During the birth it wasn't possible to bury my anger anymore and instead I swung a little too far the other way: I went from submissive to almost aggressive. It seemed some of my team members were actually a bit afraid of my new management style. It was only after the EMDR session that I finally calmed down again. I noticed big changes in my leg, arm and shoulder muscles. For the first few days I felt as if I had been run over by a bus, and had massages to allow my muscles to relax again.

The coaching sessions took me from being submissive, temporarily through a period of being aggressive, to finding a good balance of assertiveness. I now help my female team members to be assertive too. When I feel angry, I express it and calmly explain what's bothering me and what I would like to see done differently.

My new-found assertiveness has also helped me to prepare for the birth of my second child. I learned a lot about why we have pain during childbirth and was able to apply it in a practical way. Rather than hazy breathing techniques, I practised panting with my hand in a bucket of ice to figure out what really worked and didn't work for me. I also used the birth trainer to stretch my vagina and train my pelvic floor muscles. It boosted confidence when I managed to pump the balloon up to more than eight centimetres and push it out and when I found that I could bear the ice cube hand bath much better while gently humming. In the last weeks before the birth, I practised almost every day and almost got used to the 'one minute on, three minutes off' routine. I also massaged my perineum twice a day with a special oil to increase the circulation in that area and prevent tearing during the delivery. It felt good to prepare for the birth in such a practical and active way.

The coach asked, *'How do you think the baby would like to be born?'* That question hit home. She also explained that the birth serves as a sort of initiation rite that strengthens the bond between mother and baby. I myself have maintained a strong friendship with my classmates and that is partly a result of our common experience during initiation rituals at university, so the analogy was quite appropriate. It wasn't going to be fun for me or for my baby, but I expected we would both survive it and maintain a bond forever. And that's exactly what happened.

For my second birth I borrowed a TENS machine from my midwife. The machine didn't really seem to help; I only felt an itch in my lower back. I gave birth in four hours. When my husband went to remove the stickers, the machine appeared to have been on constantly instead of from time to time. And I had kept pressing on the button! Apart from that lower back itch, I hadn't been aware of it at all, but perhaps the constant electric shocks did distract me from the pain of the contractions. It doesn't matter to me anyway, I gave birth and this time I felt happy and proud instead of angry. Our youngest daughter Faye is the sunshine of our lives." (Florence, 35 years old)

The birth plan: a wish list

Research shows that realistic expectations before the birth lead to more satisfaction after the birth. For this reason, parents-to-be are encouraged to write a birth plan in preparation for the birth. This birth plan lets you tell each other (as partners) and your caregivers (midwife, gynaecologist, clinical midwife) what you would and wouldn't like to happen during your labour. This is expressly a wish list, not a requirement list. Try describing what you would like rather than a list of things you would not like to happen. The three basic psychological needs described in Chapter 1 are relevant here. Think of what you need in order to feel safe, how you can ensure that you're taken seriously during the birth, to have the room to make your own decisions, and what you need to be able to believe in yourself and your own abilities.

Labouring women are far more sensitive to atmosphere than was previously thought. The calmer the atmosphere is around the birthing woman, the better the natural birth process will progress. The role of the five senses during labour is also often underestimated. If you can ensure that whatever you see, hear, smell, feel and taste around you are things that help you to relax, you put your senses to work for you rather than against you. If you're planning a home birth it's quite easy to create the optimal atmosphere for labour – your house is already furnished to your taste. However, you can also adapt the atmosphere in a hospital or birth clinic, so that you feel "at home" in the delivery room, rather than like a visitor. You can take your own relaxing background music, and the smell of home on your own pillow or blanket can calm your nerves in the strange place that is the delivery room. You can wrap yourself in the blanket to protect yourself from everything that's going on around you. Ask your partner or someone else to massage you on the spot that needs the most attention at that particular moment. Keep your feet warm – cold feet will steer your attention away from your labour. Ask if the light in the room can be dimmed and check in advance if you'll be allowed to shower whenever you need to. Sometimes scented candles or essential oil drops are allowed in the delivery room. Make noises, sing, laugh, growl or moan if you find that it helps to bear the contractions better.

Some of my clients use extensive birth plans that they have found online and that are several pages long. Much of that information is not relevant to their own delivery, or it is information that is already obvious for the care provider. You don't need to include this information in your birth plan. It's impossible for care providers to remember birth plans that are several pages long, especially if they're looking after more than one labouring woman at a time. Therefore, try to have a compact overview of your wishes that fits on to one page at the most. Ask your care providers to take your wishes into account and to discuss with you which considerations they are making at any given moment and which interventions they want to perform according to the medical condition of the mother and child.

It's a good idea to make two plans: Plan A for if the birth goes according to your wishes, and Plan B for if it doesn't and, for example, needs to be taken over by a gynaecologist. Once again: the aim is not to try to plan out your birth point by point. That would be impossible and you will only increase your risk of being disappointed when things don't go as you had hoped. You can however, put all chances on your side by going through various "if..., then..." scenarios beforehand together with your partner and caregivers. Focus especially on the aspects that you can do something about; situations that you can make a decision about yourself.

It's important to discuss your wishes with your midwife or doctor during pregnancy as this will prevent disappointment once you're in labour. Perhaps you'd like your midwife to stay with you if your delivery is handed over to a gynaecologist and your midwife may tell you that she can't guarantee that. It's good for you to know this well in advance of the birth, so you still have time to look for an alternative, such as hiring a doula (birth coach). You and your midwife can look for solutions together for all the potential problem areas.

The good thing is that parents-to-be and healthcare providers have a common goal: a birth experience that is as positive as possible, given the medical circumstances, with as the end result, a healthy as possible baby in the arms of a healthy as possible mother. Keep this beautiful common goal in sight while discussing your wishes as well as during the birth itself.

Let your body and mind work for you

Without wanting to repeat myself, I would like to conclude this chapter and this book by setting out a few tips to prepare for your next birth:

1. **Let your brain, your senses and your body work for you instead of against you.** Ensure that you go into the experience as relaxed and well prepared as possible. The calmer you are, the less adrenaline and cortisol there will be in your body, the more the oxytocin can work to make efficient contractions and the more pain-relieving endorphins you will produce. Breathe calmly from your stomach as much as you can (see the breathing exercises described in Chapter 3).
2. **Keep actively moving around for as long as you can and change position regularly.** Try different positions to see which one works best for you at different points. Contractions can feel very different depending on whether you're sitting, on your hands and knees, leaning over the edge of the bed or an ironing board, under the shower or in a warm bed. What might feel great at one hour can be much less pleasant later on. Keep looking for the optimal position at any given moment. Your partner can help you with this.
3. **Use visualisation and affirmations.** By studying high-level athletes we know how powerful visualisation can be.

An athlete who visualises his "Golden Race" while lying down, tenses the same muscle groups as during the actual race. On a scan, the brain activity that can be seen during the visualisation is comparable to that which can be seen during the race. Most high-level athletes also make use of positive, short statements, known as affirmations. Some examples of affirmations you can use in labour are "I'm perfectly capable of giving birth", "I'm strong" or "My baby's healthy, I'm healthy, what a wonder!".

Valerie's

Long after my first child was born, I was still feeling anxious, depressed and unsure of myself. I managed to process the birth with the help of EMDR and FHER (see Chapter 7). I also worked hard to let go of my old (family) patterns and used the observation sheet (see Chapter 8) to explore my thoughts and feelings and to change my behaviour. I wanted to have another baby but sadly had two miscarriages in a row. It felt good to go back to my coach to talk about my sadness. I also did an exercise that helped me to move on from the miscarriages. When at last I became and stayed pregnant, I felt so strong, it was like I could take on the whole world.

But then, when my maternity leave started, I had another setback. I didn't have much to distract me and started brooding about the imminent birth. I started doubting myself again and felt insecure and down. I went back to my coach and together we made a list of all the things I was worried about. For each item on the list, I then found a solution. She said I could plant pitons in the mountain of fear/anxiety that I was climbing. The pitons gave me something to hold on to. For example, I went to talk to an anaesthetist. Because I'm overweight, the epidural wasn't put in properly during the first birth.

After my first child, Derrick, was born, I lost a lot of blood because the placenta didn't separate. In the end they had to put me under a general anaesthetic to remove the placenta during an operation. Derrick was admitted to the children's ward because of an infection he got from bacteria I was carrying. A few days after the birth, I got a pounding headache. The doctors said this was because I had lost so much blood, so I was given a blood transfusion and another one two days later. All that time the headache remained and made me nauseous, especially if I sat up or got out of bed. They asked me if I was afraid of leaving the hospital with my baby – as if I was making up the atrocious headache because I didn't want to go home with my baby. My self-confidence took a hit from the feeling that I was not being taken seriously and was being treated like a drama queen. Could it all just be psychological? Eventually, it was discovered that the pain was caused by a leak in my spinal cord because of the epidural. Once they began to treat that, the pain subsided within a couple of hours.

I wanted to avoid a repetition of all that awfulness, so I started planting my pitons.

Piton 1 was making a pain relief plan with the anaesthetist.

Piton 2 was the antibiotics drip that I would get just before the birth to prevent my second son, Finn, from being infected with the bacteria.

Piton 3 was about my preparation for the birth. I practised with my hand in iced water and found that grumbling and screaming were counterproductive. A cross between growling and humming in the back of my throat seemed to be the most effective, also during the actual birth. I also trained and massaged my pelvic floor muscles every day from 37 weeks onwards. This gave me confidence in my lower body and I felt well prepared for labour.

Piton 4 was about the healthcare providers. I hadn't seen my own gynaecologist at all during the first birth. There had been three different trainee gynaecologists and many different nurses. Everything was decided over my head and behind my back and I didn't want that to happen this time around. I wanted to have a plan and if it needed to be changed I wanted to be told why, what the options were and whether it was in my best interest and that of my baby. Above all, I wanted to play a part in the decision-making. The most important thing for me was to not be left alone. The hospital promised me a doula-nurse if I chose to have an induction, because that would also be easier for the anaesthetist's special pain relief plan.

Piton 5 was the planned induction. On the day of the induction, they decided first to break my waters and then to put in place the drip with the antibiotics before starting with the oxytocin drip. I felt cramps quite soon after, but they were quite bearable. The doula-nurse was wonderful. She even massaged my back and I trusted her completely. I lay on my side, very relaxed, and had absolutely no notion of time. My husband sat near my head and during the contractions I looked in his eyes and growl-hummed my way through them, just as I had practised with the iced water. My head was so preoccupied with the antibiotics drip that needed to be empty before I could start birthing my baby that I hardly paid attention to the contractions or the pain. When the bag was finally empty, the nurse said it wouldn't be long before I could start pushing. She wanted to get the baby clothes ready and warm up the cot. What?! I thought she was taking me for a ride. The anaesthetist hadn't even been called yet. Fifteen minutes later I got the urge to push. Thirty minutes after that Finn was there. I was immediately given other medicines through the drip and another 15 minutes later the placenta was delivered. It was a perfect birth, in spite of my weight. So I was capable of giving birth! This time, the week following the birth also went very well.

That second birth restored my self-image and self-confidence so much that I finally had the courage to face my biggest challenge yet. Six months after the birth, I stopped breastfeeding and went back to see my coach. With her help and that of a personal trainer I lost 25 kilos in nine months. How symbolic – this time it wasn't a pregnancy, but nine months of losing excess weight.

Marina's

STORY

After the birth, the midwife asked me a couple of times whether it had been a traumatic experience for me and if I needed extra help to process it. I found the birth difficult but not traumatic and at that time didn't feel that I needed any assistance. The first physical symptoms appeared six months later, when I went back to work. My GP couldn't explain them. A year later I was home with a burnout. When I found information online about PTSD after childbirth, I cried tears of recognition. I went to see a childbirth processing specialist who found that I had a range of PTSD symptoms.

My first pregnancy went exceptionally well, but a month before the due date, my waters broke unexpectedly. I had been on maternity leave for just a week. Neither the midwife nor the gynaecologist was able to confirm that I was losing amniotic fluid. A week later they did find a tear in the amniotic sac and I was induced the next day. I was exactly 37 weeks pregnant then. They broke my waters by the baby's head. I went to shower because I was only one centimetre dilated. While in the shower I was hit by non-stop contractions – there was no break between them. I didn't know what was happening to me. Twenty minutes later, and still in the shower, I felt that the baby was coming. I pressed the bell. The nurse came and saw that I was ready to push. I pushed for about an hour and a quarter and then our daughter Flora was born. It was a beautiful moment.

Flora was a small baby of just 2.8 kilos and she lost more than 10% of her weight in the first few days. We had to take her to the hospital for extra checks with the paediatrician. Everything was alright, but neither Flora nor I were relaxed. Flora often choked on her milk and I was afraid she was going to suffocate. The day after her appointment with the paediatrician, Flora was listless. I could hardly get her attention. It was difficult to wake her. The midwife had to come round four times that day to help with breastfeeding and eventually that was the turning point. Flora started drinking better, she began to grow and was more alert. I felt extremely responsible for her and overprotective. I even thought in that first week: if I'd known beforehand how heavy the responsibility for a baby feels, I never would have embarked on this. During a coaching session I felt that sense of responsibility again on my shoulders and pushing against my chest. The coach explained that the combination of many life events in a short period of time and traumatic experiences may have contributed to the burnout. In the space of a couple of years I had got married, we had drastically renovated our home, had moved house twice, I had got a new job and had a lot of stress at work. If you include two difficult births, you see the result: a burnout. The coaching sessions helped me to feel and accept my anxiety, overprotectiveness and sense of responsibility. To *"Feel it and Heal it"*. In addition, the focus was on relaxation. My system first had to come to rest. I saw a masseur and did relaxation exercises every day.

During one coaching session I rewound the videotape of the birth and recorded my ideal birth over it *("Erase and Replace")*. My ideal birth was much calmer than Flora's birth was in reality. I stopped working at 34 weeks, so that I could be well rested when labour began. My waters broke and it was clear to everyone straight away that they had broken. The birth went well and I helped Flora to be born myself. I felt her warm body on my own. We had eye contact immediately. In this ideal version of the birth she weighed over 3 kilos and was able to feed well from the start. There were no choking or suffocating incidents, she didn't need to be seen by the paediatrician. I felt calm and full of confidence, both in myself and in my daughter. We belonged together. What I noticed is that, since I rewrote her birth story, Flora was much less clingy and played independently more. She also stopped bothering her baby brother and coming out of her bed.

Next, there was Job's birth. Just as with Flora, my waters had broken, again due to a tear in the amniotic sac and again there was hesitation as to whether or not it was amniotic fluid. This time too, I was induced after a week, and luckily this time I was 39 weeks pregnant. I was looking forward to meeting our second child. I was relaxed and trusted my body. The trainee-gynaecologist told us she was going to break my waters. As a joke I told her to put an apron on as the midwife had said there was a lot of amniotic fluid. I had barely got my words out when my waters were broken and a tsunami of fluid came bursting out. The baby's heart rate slowed dramatically. The doctor asked me to lie down on my side. We could hear the baby's heart very soft and calm in the distance. I was given an oxygen mask over my nose and mouth. That's when the most intense moments of my life began. It was like finding myself in the middle of a film in slow-motion. The doctor was repeating: *"Emergency bell, operating team, emergency C-section, cord prolapse."* I was afraid we were going to lose our baby. I saw panic in the eyes of the doctors. Within a minute the room was full of people, a well-oiled team. I was paralysed with shock. Where was Nils? I saw my husband standing in the corner of the room. I saw the fear in his eyes. I wanted him to hold my hand but someone had just stuck a catheter into it. I felt helpless and hopeless. The doctor's hand was in my vagina all the time; I could feel her pushing the baby upwards. After that, a litre of water was pumped into my bladder to hold the baby's head in place. Suddenly the bed started moving, I was being pushed to the operating room. There was a man waiting by the lift and the doctor shouted: *"Emergency! That lift is for us!"* I was shoved into the lift. The doors closed and the bed was stuck between them. I thought: it's all over now. Suddenly Nils jumped on to the bed and pushed the lift doors open. The bed rolled into the lift and Nils fell on to the doctor who was sitting on the bed with her hand in my vagina. What an awful film it was. Luckily, the lift doors opened again at the floor of the operating room. We flew down the corridors and I watched the ceiling lights flash by. I could only think about our child. What if he didn't get enough oxygen and was brain-damaged? What would our lives be like? Before I knew what was happening, I was wheeled into the operating room. I hadn't even had time to say goodbye to Nils. The epidural was put in place and the operation began. Suddenly Nils was at my side. I was so happy to see him, I could have cried.

The baby was born and Nils went with the paediatrician. I didn't even know if it was a boy or a girl. Once the doctor had finished examining the baby, Nils came back to me together with the nurse. We have a son, he told me. The nurse laid Job for a moment with his cheek against mine and we were together for a second, the three of us. I asked if Job could stay with me, but that wasn't possible. Nils went back to the maternity ward with Job. It took an hour for them to close my wound. During that time I felt unreal and very lonely – what had just happened? I felt as though my baby and my birth had been taken away from me, even though I understood that everything was being done in his and my best interests. I was so upset that I wasn't able to hold the baby against my bare skin. I had to make do with the memory of a few seconds of feeling his warm cheek against mine.

In the recovery room I felt very sad. I was trembling and felt nauseous. The epidural had been placed too high up. When I was finally allowed in the maternity ward, I found that Job had been lying on my husband's chest all that time. That felt good. He gave Job to me, but I felt too weak and sick because of the epidural. I was still in shock and mumbled that I was afraid of dropping the baby, so they took my little one away again to wash him. I immediately felt guilty, as if I had rejected Job. Although I was still in the room I felt like I was drifting away. I only called my mother hours later to tell her what had happened. I remember almost nothing of that conversation. I couldn't sleep that night; I was so scared of losing Job. The following week was chaotic. I wasn't able to breastfeed. Everyone was extremely tense because of what had happened. I asked Nils to stay home a bit longer, but he said he didn't dare ask for more time off as it was a very busy time at work. I had the feeling that I had to beg him to do things that he had done unquestioningly before the birth. During and after Flora's birth we had been a team, we had done it together. This time I felt alone. In the end, Nils stayed home the second week. The housekeeping was taken over by my mother and mother-in-law. It was very kind of them, of course, but it added to my sense that I was losing control of my home and my life. It may sound strange but my feeling of having failed at birthing my baby was reinforced by the fact that Nils didn't give me a gift, as he had done when Flora was born. That time I had received a beautiful watch, this time I got nothing. It was as if I didn't deserve a gift because I hadn't pushed Job out myself. I had both the feeling that I had failed during the birth and that I had lost Nils during the birth.

During the EMDR session, all the emotions I had taken for granted during the birth came up, even some emotions that I had forgotten about. Rationally, I knew that I hadn't failed, but that sense was very strong during the EMDR session. I then felt enormous anger towards the doctor for breaking my waters and this feeling too faded again. It was as if I was in the operating room again and the loneliness that I had felt then came back to me. I realised at the same time that I was in my coach's office and that I was watching a kind of film, but it felt real. After the EMDR, I began to feel better. At work, however, there was very little understanding for what I had been through. They didn't see how a traumatic birth experience a year and a half earlier could lead to a burnout. I really felt let down by my work and my manager. It was so disappointing, after I had given everything to them for seven years. Eventually

I decided to take a different path and leave my job. By sharing my story in this book I hope to bring more understanding to employers and work doctors about the impact a traumatic birth can have on your life.

Nils's

The birth of our eldest child went very fast and – from my point of view – very well. It was all done and dusted within a couple of hours. If it was like this, I could have another three children! Eighteen months later, we were in the middle of major renovations and moving house when Marina was unexpectedly pregnant with our second baby. We had planned a second child but were surprised by how quickly it happened. I was busy with the renovations, Marina was busy at work (with a restructuring) and with caring for our daughter. With hindsight, it was at that point that the distance started to grow between us. At first, the second birth looked a lot like the first. Again it was unclear for a few days whether or not the waters had broken, and again the birth had to be induced. We were ready to welcome our baby and everything seemed to be going well. My wife could give birth like the best of them and I had complete faith in her and in the medical team.

The trainee-gynaecologist said she was going to break the waters. Something in me wanted to stop her, but I couldn't say: *"Don't do it, I have a bad feeling about it!"*, without any medical argument whatsoever about why it felt "bad". So I said nothing – and I blamed myself for this afterwards. If only I had stopped the doctor, I might have prevented what occurred next. The doctor broke the waters and a tidal wave of amniotic fluid gushed into the room. All hell broke loose. I saw the doctor look with panic at the nurse and heard her call "emergency". I had no idea what was happening. People were running into the room from all over. I was literally pushed into a corner. I felt helpless and hopeless. I made myself as small as possible so as not to get in anyone's way. No-one explained anything to me. I tried to make eye contact with Marina over the heads of all the medical staff. Somebody said "cord prolapse" and I thought that meant our baby was going to suffocate on the spot. The plugs were pulled out of the wall and they started running with the bed with Marina in it. The doctor was sitting on the bed, her hand inside Marina. Somebody asked: *"Are you coming?"*. I had no idea I was allowed to go with them and I ran after Marina (feeling literally and figuratively left behind).

The lift was called with an emergency button and Marina was shoved into it with the bed and the doctor. The doors got stuck around the bed – they would neither open nor close. I thought: I'm not going to let my child die because the stupid lift won't open or close. I jumped on to the bed, pushed my back against one side and my feet against the other door with all my might. The strength you find at such a moment is unbelievable. The lift doors shot open, the bed rolled in and I tumbled in after it. We ran down the corridors to the operating rooms. Someone told me: *"You can't go any further."* I saw Marina disappear into the OR and didn't know if I would see her or our son alive again. I wanted the ground to open up and swallow me. Someone else came up to me and asked: "Why haven't you got dressed yet?" I didn't understand. I was given an operating gown to wear and was taken to Marina's head. The rest of her body was hidden by light blue sheets and the C-section had already started. A few minutes later, Job was lifted up. He cried and everything seemed to be alright. He was examined by the paediatrician and I was told to go upstairs with him. It didn't feel right to leave Marina behind in the OR, but I just did as I was told, still completely in shock. Once in the room I laid Job on my bare chest. Marina had done that with our first baby and we wanted to have skin-on-skin contact with this baby too for the first hour after birth, in order to promote the breastfeeding. It felt good to have Job's warm body against mine, but I hardly dared breathe, let alone look at him. I sat as still as possible, even thought it was more than an hour and a half before Marina was back from the operating room. We looked at each other and both saw the fear in each other's eyes. What had happened to us in such a short time?

I wanted to be strong for Marina, she had just been though an operation after all. I felt tense and escaped in my work. I was so busy pushing away my feelings that I felt nothing at all anymore. Marina constantly tried to talk to me about that, but it just made me want to run away more. She became annoyed by my constant running away, I was annoyed with her wish to talk about the birth and our changed relationship and we grew further away from each other.

I had been so frightened when watching powerless in the corner of the delivery room, when I had no idea what was happening and whether my child was going to live. People asked me if the part with the lift was the worst, but on the contrary, I was able to do something there and had some added value. When I told my story to the coach, sobbing and snivelling, she noticed that my shoulders were up by my ears and that I was breathing very fast. She asked if I had been holding my breath, in a sense, since the birth. Coincidentally, just the week before, I had been referred by the GP to a cardiologist because of a stifling feeling and had been diagnosed with hyperventilation.

In that same coaching session I redid the birth using the FHER method. In my version, the onset of labour was calm and spontaneous, the waters broke only when Marina was fully dilated, there was a sense of calm in the delivery room and, just as we had done with our daughter, we birthed the baby together. The coach said softly that I could take the baby, if I wanted to, and that was a very special moment. I could feel him in my hands. This time I was able to look at Job from all angles before laying him on Marina's chest. I whispered to him: *"Welcome, dear Job. I'm your Daddy and I'm going to keep you safe."* The tears streamed down my face – it was so beautiful and it felt so "real". I took Job on to my chest, this time breathing evenly. It felt "right". My heart was beating calmly, Job was calm, Marina was calm and the birth had happened calmly. We had done it together. I left the coach's office and felt as if I had left my heavy winter coat behind.

After that session I went to see a breathing therapist. It was still a few months before my breathing was completely back to normal.

Marina and Nils's

Marina: After we had both processed the traumatic birth of our second child individually, we went together for a final session with the coach. We had really lost each other a bit since the birth of our little boy. When our daughter was born, we were really a team; for our son, we had both felt alone. Because we had processed our unpleasant birth experience separately, we could relate better to each other's experience. Nils understood that I had felt misunderstood and unsupported and I understood that his behaviour was a result of fear and not of lack of interest. We had both been afraid but dealt with it each in our own way. Nils fell back on caring for Flora in the first few days. He wanted her life to continue as normally as possible. I saw that he wasn't feeling good and he saw that I wasn't feeling good, but we couldn't reach each other and were both in survival mode. We got irritated by one another. Nils hadn't told me before that he had felt so strongly for the doctor not to break my waters. I hadn't realised that he didn't know what was happening while he was standing in the corner, because the doctor did explain it to me. Thanks to this talk we were able to put our stories together. We had both felt helpless and hopeless, when it suddenly became very hectic in the delivery room after the waters were broken. I found it special to hear that the moment in the lift was much more positive for Nils than for me, because he was finally able to actively do something to help.

Nils: It felt good that Marina understood how much I wanted to protect her, and wanted to spare her and Job the C-section, but that I hadn't been able to do so. The coach explained that fear had put me in the *freeze*-mode during the birth and then into a *flight*-mode once Marina was home again. I wanted to do things differently but I was incapable. It felt good to finally make this clear to her. It confirmed what she had felt all along. It was also good to be able to tell her the operation part from my point of view; how at first I wasn't allowed in, then I was with her for a while and then had to go with Job and leave her alone. It felt as though I had chosen the side of my child over my wife. When Marina said how happy she had been to find out that Job had lain on my chest all that time and that she was grateful to me for that, it felt good. Apparently I had done something right. I really needed that approval from her.

Marina: It was nice that Nils understood that I missed him, that I needed him, because he was the only familiar face in all that chaos. The coach asked us to redo that part of the story, as if we had been able to be together, just the three of us, after the birth. Instinctively we touched our heads together. I felt again Job's warm cheek against mine and at the same time, Nils's arms around me. I felt safe and connected to Nils. I told him how anxious and lonely I had been in the recovery room and how sick I had felt when I was back in the ward... how painful it was for me to be too sick to hold Job in my arms.

Nils: I thought you were having an epileptic fit, you were lying shaking in bed with your eyes rotating. It was terrifying! I was afraid of losing you too. You wanted to talk about it, I couldn't talk about it. So I focused on my work and on Flora, at least I could do that. I hated that we were always fighting, because we almost never did before Job was born – we usually understood each other without even needing to speak.

Marina: This might be really silly, but after Flora was born you gave me that beautiful watch as a gift. It felt like a sort of recognition for my effort when she was born. After Job was born, I didn't get anything from you and felt as though you thought I didn't perform well at the birth. I missed having that gift as a symbol of your recognition.

Nils: Oh, darling, I didn't buy you a gift because I didn't want a piece of jewellery to remind you of the nightmare of the birth. I did think about it a few times, but it didn't feel right, not even for myself, to buy something that would remind us of that day. You did amazingly well and you are a wonderful mother to our children.

Marina and Nils: After the session we walked away armed for the future. After more than a year and a half, we felt connected again on a deeper level. We make an effort now to go out together again and our relationship is as solid as it was before Job was born. We're very happy that we could process the birth, first separately, and then together.

Acknowledgments

I cannot thank the twenty-six members of my think tank enough for their indispensable feedback. In the most impossible week of the year, between the Christmas dinner and the New Year parties of 2015, you found the time to read this book critically and – working from your own individual areas of expertise – to dot the i's and cross the t's. Amongst other things, I received feedback from a mountain top in Switzerland, a pep-talk from a French retreat and a Christmas 'writing-means-cutting' Skype conversation from Rome. I am grateful for your involvement and genuine engagement with the subject that is so close to my heart: Mieke Lambregtse-van den Berg and Sascha Kats (psychiatrists); Ineke de Kruijff and Carole Lasham (paediatricians); Cora Harteveld and José Stolk (infant mental health specialists); Inge van Kamp, Renske Dullemond, Claire Stramrood and Els Dufraimont (gynaecologists); Katinka de Wijs and Tosca Gort (psychologists); Marjan Sepers (EMDR specialist); Sara van Marle-Jeurissen (general practitioner); Antoinette Kuiper-van der Meché and Angelique Verstegen (delivery procedures specialists); Sabrina Boekhoud and Gerdien Raasveld (experiential experts); Els Schepens (psychotherapist); Yvonne Fontein-Kuipers and Lilian Wirken (midwives); Jeannette Rietberg and Daan Westerink (grief specialists); Karin Wagenaar (Emotionally Focused Therapy (EFT) specialist); Jacqueline van Gent (Transactional Analysis (TA) specialist). Together, we can break the taboo surrounding birth trauma by creating a multidisciplinary approach, and not least because of your passion and ability to think from the heart.

Marlijn Visser, obstetrician, coach, delivery procedures specialist, think tank member and, above all, a dear friend: thank you for your Apps and prayers when I needed them most. Your unconditional support throughout the writing process has been invaluable.

Niek de Bruijn: the dedication at the front of this book describes only a fraction of what you mean to me. I'm grateful for your support: as my partner, as a perfect father (who does exist!) to Tess and Bregje, as my best friend, critic, sounding board, chef, website builder, PowerPoint maker and designer. I hope that we'll stay together forever (as lovers, parents, friends and colleagues).

Katrien Van Oost: 'perfect' publishers also exist! Thank you for your encouragement, mentoring, patience, trust, critical eye and linguistic brilliance. I appreciate your kindness and for being available at evenings and weekends. This book kept me occupied 24/7 and I expected the same of you.

Dik Klut: I am thrilled that you also wanted to illustrate my second book. Your ability to capture the essence of each chapter in a single image fills me with wonder. Thank you for your patience and your endless creative quest to find the 'perfect' cover for this publication. Dear clients: thank you for your openness, for exposing your vulnerabilities and for your trust. Daring to share such profound and intimate childbirth experiences is nothing short of brave. Through your taboo-breaking accounts that others can identify with, you provide recognition and support for parents who have experienced childbirth as an all-encompassing and life-changing event.

Above all, your stories convey the love you feel for your children. I hope that this will inspire other parents to seek the help they need to process their own experiences of childbirth, for the sake of themselves and their children. Finally, I hope your testimonies stimulate caregivers to reflect, from a client's perspective, upon their own actions and ways of communicating during childbirth.

Bibliography

Adams, S. et al (2012). *Fear of Childbirth and duration of labour: a study of 2206 women with intended vaginal delivery.* British Journal of Obstetrics and Gynaecology, 119 (10): 1238-1246.

Alder, J. et al (2007). *Depression and anxiety during pregnancy: a risk factor for obstetric, fetal and neonatal outcome? A critical review of the literature.* Journal of Maternal-Fetal and Neonatal Medicine, 20(3): 189-209.

Andersson, L. et al (2004). *Neonatal outcome following maternal antenatal depression and anxiety: a population-based study.* American Journal of Epidemiology, 159 (9): 872-881.

Ayers, S. (2008). *Post-traumatic stress disorder following childbirth: current issues and recommendations for future research.* Journal of Psychosomatic Obstetrics & Gynaecology, 29(4): 240-250.

Balkom, A.L.J.M. van, et al (2013). *Multidisciplinaire Richtlijn Angststoornissen.* Utrecht, Trimbos Instituut/GGZ-richtlijnen.

Bennet, H.A. et al (2004). *Prevalence of depression during pregnancy: systematic review.* Journal of Obstetrics and Gynaecology, 103(4): 689-709.

Berg, M.P. van den (2006). *Parental Psychopathology and the early developing child - Generation R study.* Proefschrift Erasmus Universiteit Rotterdam.

Bergh, B.R. et al (2005). *Antenatal maternal anxiety and stress and the neurobehavioural development of the fetus and child: links and possible mechanisms. A review.* Journal of Neuroscience & Biobehavioral Reviews, 29(2): 237-258.

Bergink, V. (2012). *First-onset postpartum psychosis.* Proefschrift Erasmus Universiteit Rotterdam.

Bijl, R.C. et al. (2016). *A retrospective study on persistent pain after childbirth in the Netherlands.* Journal of Pain Research, 9: 1-8.

Boelens, W (2012). *Behandelprotocol Depressie.* Amsterdam, Uitgeverij Boom.

Brockington, I.F. et al (2006). *The Post Partum Bonding Questionnaire: a validation.* Archives of Womens Mental Health, 9(5): 233-242.

Broeke, E. ten, Jongh, A. de (2009). *Praktijkboek EMDR, casusconceptualisatie en specifieke doelgroepen.* Amsterdam, Uitgeverij Pearson.

Buckle, J. (2004). *Parental devastation and regeneration following the death of a child.* Dissertation Abstracts International: Section B: The Sciences and Engineering, 64 (8-B): 4025 e.v.

Clason, E. (2011). *Babypraat.* Baarn, Forte Uitgevers.

Corbeil, M. et al (2015). *Singing delays the onset of infant distress.* Infancy, doi: 10.1111/infa.12144.

Crowley, S.K. et al (2012). *Efficacy of light therapy for perinatal depression: a review.* Journal of Physiological Anthropology, doi: 10.1186/1880-6805-31-15.

Deci, E. L., et al (2013). *'Self-determination theory and actualization of human potential',* in: D. McInerney, H. Marsh, R. Craven, & F. Guay (eds.), *Theory driving research: New wave perspectives on self processes and human development;* 109-133.

Diekstra, R. F. W. (2006). *Ik kan denken/voelen wat ik wil.* Amsterdam, Uitgeverij Pearson.

Ejegård. H, et al. (2008). *Sexuality after Delivery with Episiotomy: A Long-Term Follow-up.* Gynecologic and Obstetric Investigation, 66: 1-7.

Fontein, Y. (2016). *WazzUp Mama?! The development of an intervention to prevent and reduce maternal distress during pregnancy.* Proefschrift Universiteit van Maastricht.

Fontein, Y. et al (2014). *Antenatal interventions to reduce maternal distress: a systematic review and meta-analysis of randomised trials.* British Journal of Obstetrics and Gynaecology, 121(4): 389-397.

Hengeveld, M.W. (2014). Handboek voor de classificatie van psychische stoornissen DSM-5. Amsterdam, Uitgeverij Boom.

Holmes, E.A. et al (2007). Imagery rescripting in cognitive behaviour therapy: images, treatment techniques and outcomes. Journal of Behavior Therapy and Experimental Psychiatry, 38(4): 297-305.

Hornsveld, H., Berendsen, S. (red) (2009). Casusboek EMDR. Houten, Uitgeverij Bohn Stafleu van Loghum.

Hout, M.A. van den (2012). *Tones inferior to eye movements in the EMDR treatment of PTSD.* Behavior Research and Therapy, 50(5): 275-279.

Hout, M.A. van den, Engelhard, I. (2012). *How does EMDR work?* Journal of Experimental Psychopathology, 3(5): 724-738.

Johnson, S. (2008). *Hold me tight.* New York, Little, Brown.

Jongh, A. de, Broeke, E. ten (2009). *Handboek EMDR, een geprotocolleerde behandelmethode voor de gevolgen van psychotrauma.* Amsterdam, Uitgeverij Pearson.

Kamm, S., Vandenberg B. (2001). *Grief communication, grief reactions and marital satisfaction in bereaved parents.* Death Studies, 25(7): 569-582.

Karp, H. (2003). *The happiest baby on the block.* New York, Bantam Books.

Korrelboom, C.W., Broeke, E. ten (2004). *Handboek Geïntegreerde cognitieve gedragstherapie.* Bussum, Uitgeverij Coutinho.

Koster, D. (2012). *Perfecte moeders bestaan niet. Het boek dat zwangere vrouwen en moeders helpt in balans te komen en te blijven.* Tielt, Uitgeverij Lannoo.

Koster, D. (2014). *Impact en gevolgen van een traumatische baring.* Tijdschrift voor Verloskundigen, 4: 54-57.

Krakow, B. et al (1995). *Imagery rehearsal treatment for chronic nightmares.* Behaviour Research and Therapy, 33(7): 837-843.

Lambregtse-van den Berg, M. et al (2015). *Handboek psychiatrie en zwangerschap.* Utrecht, Uitgeverij de Tijdstroom.

Lapp, L.K. et al (2010). *Management of post traumatic stress disorder after childbirth: a review.* Journal of Psychosomatic Obstetrics & Gynecology, 31(3): 113-122.

Lasham, C. (2014). *De Karp-methode.* Utrecht, Kosmos Uitgevers.

Meaney, M.J. en Szyf, M. *Environmental programming of stress responses through DNA methylation: life at the interface between a dynamic environment and a fixed genome.* Dialogues in Clinical Neuroscience, 7(2): 103-123.

Meissner, B.R. (2011). *Emotionale Narben aus Schwangerschaft und Geburt auflösen: Mutter-Kind-Bindungen heilen oder unterstützen.* Meissner Verlag.

Puyvelde, M. van et al (2014), *Shall we dance? Music as a port of entrance to maternal-infant intersubjectivity in a context of postnatal depression,* Infant Mental Health Journal, 35(3); 220-232.

Rexwinkel, M. et al (2011). *Handboek Infant Mental Health.* Assen, Uitgeverij Koninklijke Van Gorcum.

Rietberg, J. i.s.m. Pel, M. (2013). *Altijd een kind te kort.* Uitgeverij Dair.

Rosenberg, M.B. (2015). *Nonviolent Communication: A Language of Life,* 3rd Edition. Encinitas, PuddleDancer Press.

Ruckhäberle, E. et al (2009). *Prospective randomized multicentre trial with the birth trainer EPI-NO® for the prevention of perineal trauma.* Australian and New Zealand Journal of Obstetrics and Gynecology, 49(5): 478-83.

Rytwinski, N.K. et al (2013). *The co-occurrence of major depressive disorder among individuals with posttraumatic stress disorder: a meta-analysis.* Journal of Traumatic Stress, 26(3): 299-309.

Sandström, M. et al (2006). *A pilot study of eye movement desensitisation and reprocessing treatment (EMDR) for post-traumatic stress after childbirth.* Midwifery, 24(1): 62-73.

Shapiro, F., Silk Forrest, M. (2005). *EMDR: The Breakthrough Therapy for Overcoming Anxiety, Stress, and Trauma.* New York, Basic Books.

Shapiro, F. (1989). *Eye Movement Desensitization: A new treatment for Post-Traumatic Stress Disorder (PTSD).* Journal of Behavior Therapy and Experimental Psychiatry, 20(3): 211-217.

Shapiro, F. (1996), *Eye Movement Desensitization and Reprocessing (EMDR): Evaluation of controlled PTSD research.* Journal of Behavior Therapy and Experimental Psychiatry, 27(3): 290-218.

Slagboom, M. (2011). *Echo. Prenataal onderzoek en keuzevrijheid.* Amsterdam, Uitgeverij Augustus.

Söderquist, J. et al (2009). *Risk factors in pregnancy for post-traumatic stress and depression after childbirth.* British Journal of Obstetrics and Gynaecology, 116(5): 672-680.

Spoormaker, V.I., Bout, J. van den (2006). *Lucid dreaming treatment for nightmares: a pilot study.* Psychotherapy and Psychosomatics, 75 (6): 389-394.

Stramrood, C.A.I. (2013). *Posttraumatic stress following pregnancy and childbirth.* Proefschrift Rijksuniversiteit Groningen.

Stramrood, C.A.I. et al (2011). *Posttraumatic stress disorder following preeclampsia and PPROM: a prospective study with 15 months follow-up.* Reproductive Sciences, 18(7): 645-653.

Stramrood, C.A.I. et al (2012). *The patient observer: eye-movement desensitization and reprocessing for the treatment of posttraumatic stress following childbirth.* Birth, 39(1): 70-76.

Stroebe, M., Schut. H. (1999). *The dual process model of coping with bereavement: rationale and description.* Death Studies, 23(3): 197-224.

Surkan, P J. et al (2009). *Social support after stillbirth for prevention of maternal depression.* Acta Obstetricia et Gynecologica Scandinavica, 88 (12): 1358-1364.

Thunnissen, M., Graaf, A. de (2013). *Leerboek Transactionele Analyse.* Utrecht: Uitgeverij De Tijdstroom.

Toller, P., Braithwaite D. (2009). *Grieving together and apart: bereaved parents' contradictions of marital interaction.* Journal of Applied Communication Research, 37(3): 257-277.

Veringa, I., Cranenburgh, B. van (2010). *Baringspijn is er niet voor niets.* Medisch Contact, 65(36): 1734-1737.

Verweij, R. en Bakel, H.J.A. van (2007). *Hongeren naar huidcontact.* Medisch Contact 62(31-32); 1319-1321.

Wijma, K. et al (1997). *Posttraumatic stress disorder after childbirth: a cross sectional study.* Journal of Anxiety Disorders, 11(6): 587-597.

Wijma, K. (1998). *Psychometric aspects of the WDEQ; a new questionnaire for the measurement of fear in childbirth.* Journal of Psychosomatic Obstetrics and Gynaecology, 19(2): 84-97.

Wirken, L. (2015). *Als bevallen spannend is. Met vertrouwen in verwachting.* Uitgeverij Forcean.